IMMUNIZATION

■

The ills from which we are suffering have had
their seat in the very foundation of human thought.

—Teilhard de Chardin

IMMUNIZATION

■

THE REALITY
BEHIND
THE MYTH

■

WALENE JAMES

FOREWORD BY ROBERT S. MENDELSOHN, M.D.

BERGIN & GARVEY
New York • Westport, Connecticut • London

Library of Congress Cataloging-in-Publication Data

James, Walene.
  Immunization: the reality behind the myth.

  Bibliography: p.
  Includes index.
  1. Immunization—Complications and sequelae.
2. Immunization of children—Complications and
sequelae. 3. National immunity. 4. Alternative
medicine. I. Title.
RA638.J34 1988   614.4'7   88-4283
ISBN 0-89789-155-4 (alk. paper)
ISBN 0-89789-154-6 (pbk.: alk. paper)

Library of Congress Catalog Card Number: 88-4283
ISBN: 0-89789-155-4
      0-89789-154-6 (pbk.)

First published in 1988

Bergin & Garvey, One Madison Avenue, New York, NY 10010
An imprint of Greenwood Publishing Group, Inc.

Printed in the United States of America

The paper used in this book complies with the
Permanent Paper Standard issued by the National
Information Standards Organization (Z39.48-1984).

10 9 8 7 6 5 4 3 2

To awakening people everywhere
May your choices be conscious

C O N T E N T S

■

PREFACE

There is an old Zen saying: "Family treasure doesn't come in through the front gate." Not a few have observed that that which intrudes upon us through the media is least valuable, and that which has real value is usually hidden or, at least, must be searched for. The information in this book is not information that "comes in through the front gate." Mainstream media, schools, and doctors will not give you this information. Most of the time they don't know it. My own search for, and discovery of, this knowledge has continued for over 35 years.

I began taking notes for this book on August 19, 1981, when the state, in the person of a social worker, rang our doorbell and informed us that a member of our family, a young person in excellent health, was required by law to submit to a medical procedure which is not only fraught with risk but is not even guaranteed to be effective. I am speaking, of course, of immunization. The story of that encounter and its aftermath—including three court hearings—is told in Chapters 9 and 10. Because tape recorders weren't allowed in court, I wrote down what happened immediately afterwards. The story in these two chapters is taken from a diary I kept during that period and from notes I kept of important encounters during the next few years.

Because the case received considerable publicity, both local and national, I found myself besieged with requests for information on the subject of childhood immunizations. I discovered people were starving for information; they were looking for something more than propaganda and the official line given them by their pediatricians and their health departments. Part I of this book, Chapters 1 through 4, was written in response to this need. It explores some of the mythology of immunization—its vaunted safety, effectiveness, and responsibility for the decline of infectious diseases—and suggests other more natural ways of creating immunity.

The more I talked with people, however, the more I realized the need for reorientation, for a more salutary and liberating way of thinking about our bodies and the microorganismic life outside and within them. It is not enough to hand people reports of the degree of harmfulness and/or ineffectiveness of specific vaccines and have them leave hoping for better ones to come down the pike. The fear of the unknown, the "dread" disease, is still there, and the weighing of the dangers of the vaccine versus the dangers of the disease still haunts them. Hence, Part II of this book.

Part II, Chapters 5 through 8, explores the subject of immunization on a deeper level—its theoretical premises, the germ theory of disease, disease seen from other perspectives, and the mental-emotional-aesthetic implications of a particular health care philosophy. Chapter 5, the most technical and a pivotal chapter in the book, tells of a little-known controversy between two scientists that took place over 100 years ago and subsequent research that supports the findings of one of these scientists, a man unknown to most of us. If his discoveries and their implications had become "establishment," the world would be a far healthier place to live, and health care would be a fraction of its present cost. And there would be no immunizations.

Part III, Chapters 9 through 12, deals with the implications of a monolithic, coercive health care system for a democratic society. Chapters 9 and 10 tell what happened to us when we tried to say, "No thank you," to the system. Others have told similar stories.

Because we are immersed in a sea of communications media—and are living in a "moneytheistic" technocracy —propaganda and misinformation are primary facts of life. Nowhere is this better illustrated than in the area of immunization. Therefore, I included a chapter on propaganda and general semantics as applied to health care. If we are to mature as individuals and as a nation, we need to develop perceptiveness and discrimination. Recognizing propaganda and misinformation is part of this process. In the health care field it can be a matter of health or disability and even life or death. "If humanity is to pass safely through its present crisis on earth," Buckminster Fuller reminds us, "it will be because a majority of individuals are now doing their own thinking" This chapter and, indeed, this book is a step in that direction.

Chapter 12 projects us into a multi-optioned, open-ended health care system, bringing together much of what has been implied throughout the book. As you may well imagine, this book steps on some very big toes. If a fraction of what its pages contains is taken seriously by enough people, enormous vested ego and economic interests stand to lose. But decay provides fertile soil for new life, aiding the transformation of old paradigms into new ones.

At the least, this book will be controversial. But what is controversy? The word itself comes from Latin and means "turned opposite." That which is controversial is turned opposite a dominating structure, in this case, establishment medicine. In a free and open society, there would be no such label as "controversial," only disagreement within an open forum of ideas and options. There would be no one mainstream, but many streams, each meeting different needs.

A word about myself: Beyond a few chemistry, physics, and biology courses, my formal education has been concentrated in the liberal arts. I taught English in the Los Angeles high schools for seven years. This I consider an advantage, because, not being a health care professional, I don't have years of indoctrination in a particular point of view to unlearn, nor do I have a job or a license that can be threatened for speaking out. The late John Holt, a leading humanistic educator, took pride in pointing out that he never took an education course. He felt he had the advantage of not having his perceptions clouded with a lot of preconceptions—and misconceptions.

About some of the challenges in writing this book: (1) The biggest challenge, of course, was making difficult, technical material easy and interesting to read. To that end I have defined technical terms when I needed to use them; however, I have used as little medical terminology as possible, retaining just enough to give the reader a sense of authenticity and the flavor of "medicalese." (2) Although I point out some of the fallacies of relying on statistics to support an argument, I use them. Why? Because they are a tool, and numbers still impress people. I have tried, however, to use just enough cases to make my point, though many more could be cited. (3) Because of the "sensitive" positions of some of the people referred to in this book, I was not given permission to use their names and have used either a fictitious name (so designated) or have simply referred to them as a "woman," a "doctor," etc. (4) I did not attempt to write the proverbial "balanced" exposition. The "other side" is so available, so much a part of our culture that to give it more quarter in a book of this nature would be superfluous.

Because my purpose in writing this book was not to fill minds as much as to open them, the focus is on principles rather than details and technical minutiae. Unless data and ideas resonate against a background of larger principles, they remain small and inert, unable to pass beyond the single track of thesis-antithesis. It is this field of larger principles that must be brought into focus before the facts within it can be given life and thus become part of a living culture. Bringing these unifying principles into focus facilitates consciousness raising. To this end this book was written.

FOREWORD

Immunization: The Reality Behind the Myth is just that! Of course, it provides the most up-to-date, completely and authoritatively documented, comprehensive critique of vaccines. From Pasteur's smallpox scam to vaccine-linked AIDS, Walene James's book is the state-of-the-art statement on vaccine damage. And its early chapters should legitimately terrify every parent whose child faces immunizations as well as everyone who already has been so victimized.

But, true to its title, *Immunization* delivers far more than a scientific indictment of the "holy water" of Modern Medicine's idolatrous, deadly religion. Walene James leads us through the matrix of modern medical mistakes responsible for the blind acceptance of vaccines. She introduces readers to unknown scientists including Bechamp and Virchow who provide the antidote to the germ theory of disease.

And beyond that, James offers sensible advice to those who already have been damaged. Not content with only destroying old myths, she provides optimism and hope by her common-sense prescriptions for wise, healthful living.

Elegance of style is an additional bonus. For example, James compares modern vaccines—laden with formaldehyde, mercury, dog kidney tissue—with the "eye of newt and toe of frog" added to the brew of Macbeth's witches. She wisely comments: "Is it too impudent to suggest that man has long had a love affair with decomposing animal proteins, noxious potions that ward off the demons of ill fortune?"

Immunization: The Reality Behind the Myth will open the eyes of those who still believe in the religion of modern medicine. It will strengthen those who have left that religion. And to protect every human being right from the start—this book is the most valuable gift you can present to the mother of a newborn baby.

ROBERT S. MENDELSOHN, M.D.
AUTHOR, *Confessions of a Medical Heretic*

ACKNOWLEDGMENTS

I wish to express my appreciation to the following:

My daughter Tanya and my grandson Isaac, whose confrontation with the Virginia Beach courts provided the impetus for writing this book.

Clinton Miller of the National Health Federation, whose advice and moral support during the litigation process and whose encouragement during the early drafts of the manuscript were invaluable.

My daughter Ingri, whose sustained interest and insistence that this material reach people helped keep me going.

Dr. Robert S. Mendelsohn, courageous pioneer in awakening the public from the harmful but lucrative superstitions of modern medicine, for writing the Foreword.

Jim Bergin, publisher; Ann Gross, editor; and the rest of the staff at Bergin & Garvey for their valuable suggestions and professional handling of the manuscript.

The late Dr. Gina Cerminara for her beginning and advanced courses in General Semantics, and Alice Lynton of the Los Angeles City School Districts Division of Secondary Education for the section on critical reading and propaganda in Operational Aid R63, September 1963.

The many wonderful people who contributed material for this book, especially: Dr. Michael MacLean, Joseph Nuccio, Paul Johnson, Clinton Miller, Heidi-Rose Dane, Sue Eldredge, Adella Scott Wilson, Robin Jackson, and Victoria Heasley.

And finally to my husband Paul, who edited and midwifed this book. Without his continuing guidance and encouragement it is doubtful that this book would have been born.

NOTE TO THE READER

Who has not dreamed of a disease-free world? The fountain of youth and eternal wellness have been one of the perennial dreams of humankind. The question this book poses is, "Does our present course of action—the proliferation of disease categories, disease specialists, and disease technologies such as drugs and vaccines—bring us closer to the realization of this dream?" Or is it realizable?

Immunization was chosen as the focus of this book partly because it epitomizes our present fragmented, adversarial approach to understanding and relating to disease processes. But for many readers the greatest value of this book will be its elucidation of ways to think about and respond to "disease-scare" and how to answer the question, "Should we have our child immunized?"

PART I

■

DEPROGRAMMING

Those who lack all idea that it is possible to be
wrong can learn nothing except know-how.

GREGORY BATESON, *Mind and Nature*

1

■

THE TYRANNY
OF WHAT EVERYONE
KNOWS*

*Any action that is dictated by fear or by
coercion of any kind ceases to be moral.*

MAHATMA GANDHI, *Ethical Religion*

UBIQUITY AND ADDICTION

Our age has been called the Information Age. It could also be called
the Misinformation Age. With the advent of electronic technology it is
now possible to inform/misinform more people than at any time in
history. Embedded in the bits and pieces of information/misinformation
with which we are bombarded are parts of the larger continent of "what
everyone knows," the conventional wisdom of the culture that philos-
ophers call "premises" or "basic assumptions." Because this conventional wisdom shapes and even determines our perceptions and
interpretations of the world, we might say that "what everyone knows"
sits in the control room of our collective psyche. Its power derives largely

*Title of an article in *Network Review*, Sept. 1984.

3

from our unconsciousness of it; therefore, reexamining "what everyone knows" is part of the process of becoming conscious and empowered human beings.

In our culture healing and health have become practically synonymous with the practice of medicine and its administration of drugs, surgery, radiation, and vaccination. This last ritual is the focus of this book. It was chosen because: (1) of a personal confrontation with the compulsory immunization laws of the state of Virginia; (2) of all the practices of modern medicine, this "sacrament" is the most blindly and aggressively pursued; and (3) the assumptions upon which this practice is based are the same assumptions behind much of the destructiveness and wastefulness of modern medicine. This destructiveness and wastefulness extend far beyond the parameters of medicine itself.

So ubiquitous has medical enterprise and rubric become that it is difficult to open a newspaper or magazine without encountering some article eulogizing some aspect of technological medicine—e.g., medical advice; medical "breakthroughs"; melodramas of disease and disability in which modern technological medicine comes to the rescue; organ transplants; futuristic projections involving exotic technology such as cloning, cryonics, etc. Even the problems of medically oriented health care, such as skyrocketing costs, are discussed as though the real problems were peripheral, e.g., gouging billing practices, fee splitting, unnecessary operations, incompetent surgeons, etc. Does it ever occur to us that the real problem might be within the medical system itself, its basic premises concerning the nature of man and, specifically, his relation to the conditions of health and disease? Because of the monopolistic position of the medical profession in our present health care system, these premises are firmly embedded in our culture.

When we think of a doctor, particularly a family doctor, the image of a medical doctor automatically comes to mind. Is this because only the medical model of health and disease is taught in public institutions and carried in the media? Is it because only medical doctors are permitted to be public health officers and, with few exceptions, only a medical doctor's professional opinion is recognized in a court of law? Or is it because only drug-oriented research is supported by taxpayer's money, and drugs, the right hand of modern medicine, are seen as the panacea for most of our ills? From cancer to rape, the drug answer is heralded and sought. Like the great flood, the medico-drug consciousness inundates most of the civilized world and the immunization ritual is, for most of us, our initiation into lifelong addiction to the medico-drug establishment.

"Remaining unimmunized for childhood diseases is a risk no child should face," reads a folder from the Virginia State Department of Health. The same folder also tells us that "health experts warn that unless more young children are immunized, widespread epidemics could take place once again."[1] "Epidemics are certain to occur if the immunity level of the population is not maintained by immunizing children," reads another folder from the Virginia health department.[2] Still another folder features grotesque cartoons personifying "Dangerous Childhood Diseases." We see "Mean-ole Measles," "Dippie Diphtheria," and "Locky Lockjaw" grimacing at us when we open the folder. The caption next to "Rolly Polio," who is sitting in a wheelchair holding up one of his crutches, tells us: "See that you and everyone around you has taken the oral polio vaccine." "Whoopy Whooping Cough," "Dippie Diphtheria," and "Locky Lockjaw" remind us to get booster shots, to return periodically for that all-important "protection." "Everyone, 1 year to 101 years needs a booster every 10 years," Dippy Diphtheria reminds us.[3] Other folders from the health department describe the seriousness and high fatalities of specific childhood diseases. The number of children permanently damaged by immunizations is minuscule, they assure us, and a small price to pay for that "protection" that has all but "wiped out" these terrible scourges.

"Thanks to vaccination, smallpox has been virtually banished from the globe—a triumph of a historic public-health crusade," reads an editorial in our local newspaper. This same editorial urges the state legislature to "immunize immunizations" from legal loopholes that would allow a child to "escape" immunizations because of parental objection. It points out how "measles and measles encephalitis are now on the defensive in the United States—a situation directly attributable to mass immunization of the young." Again we are reminded that "whenever an epidemic of a childhood disease occurs, the outbreak is nearly always traceable to a falloff in inoculations."[4]

Again, the power of vaccines to rescue us from the scourge of "dread" disease is eulogized: "Elena Jenkins, 10, owes her life to a new vaccine," reads a picture caption in a recent article titled "How Vaccines May End Infections Forever."[5] "Expanded immunization—using newly improved vaccines" will "prevent the six main immunizable diseases from killing an estimated 5 million children a year and disabling 5 million more," James Grant, executive director of UNICEF tells us.[6]

New vaccines and vaccine technology are further heralded: "Pioneering doctor predicts 1 vaccine for several diseases."[7] An article in the *Washington Post* is titled: "Unborn Children Can be Immunized Via the Mother."[8] And from the front page of our local newspaper: "Scientists hail new chickenpox vaccine."[9]

And so the wisdom of the culture broadcasts that disease is an unmitigated evil, a dangerous enemy that must be attacked and destroyed. Vaccines are miracle weapons that rout the invaders and save us from being conquered by them. They are one of the heroes in man's eternal struggle against the terrifying threat of disease, disability, and death.

UBIQUITY AND COERCION

"The children, kicking and screaming, were taken away from the parents and given smallpox vaccinations."[10]

"Our three school age children were suspended from a local public school district in Arkansas . . . for breaking the state immunization law. . . . The judge, without deliberation, pronounced Stephen [the father] guilty of truancy and fined him $750 plus court costs and appeal fees."[11]

A hundred years ago penalties were more severe. The mandatory vaccination law was enforced "with the threat of prison as well as the seizure of goods of persons refusing to comply."[12]

Here in Virginia the front page of our local newspaper reminds us: "No shots, no school. Students who can't prove they have been immunized against contagious childhood diseases shouldn't expect to start school Monday."[13]

It's tough to argue with ubiquity, especially when it is armed with the police powers of the state. If a parent objects to his child being vaccinated, officialdom assures him that the benefits outweigh the risks. If he persists in his refusal, he is told he is putting his child in jeopardy. Finally, if pressure doesn't work, coercion often will. If "right" is obvious and unequivocal, then forcing the "right" on others is doing them and society a service.

Has the medical-pharmaceutical industry become the state sanctioned church? A number of writers have noted the similarity of the medical profession to a priesthood and have observed that medicine and government are as interlocked today as were the church and state during the Middle Ages. For example, Drs. Robert Mendelsohn and Thomas Szasz refer to the "church of Modern Medicine" and the "therapeutic state" respectively. Dr. Szasz notes the similarity of the therapeutic state to the theocratic state of the Middle Ages. Is history doomed to repeat itself? Do the evils we think we have abolished in one age return in a different guise in another?

When ubiquity reigns, a culture becomes stuck in a stance, and interpretations of reality that are at variance with the dominant stance are locked out. For instance, in recent Congressional hearings on vaccinations—S. 2117—Congress refused to let scientists opposed to vaccinations testify before the committee.[14] Dare we open the door and ask some unthinkable questions? Let's try a few of them:

Is it possible that vaccinations might not be such a good idea? Is it possible that the premises upon which they are based might be faulty? Is it possible that the decline of infectious diseases might have little or nothing to do with the near universal practice of vaccination? Is it possible that the increase in chronic and degenerative disease is related to the parallel increase in the practice of mass vaccination?

To answer "yes" to any of these questions is to invite vigorous opposition and defensiveness from the medical community. Because of its enormous investment—ego as well as monetary—in this practice, this community will resist answers that threaten its image and position. The door to discovery, however, is opened by knowing how to ask the right questions and by not being afraid to look at the answers.

NOTES

1. "Protect them from harm," Virginia State Department of Health, Richmond. I picked up the literature from the health department on Independence Boulevard in Virginia Beach, summer 1982.
2. "Questions and Answers on Polio," Virginia State Department of Health, Richmond.
3. "Parents—State Law Requires . . . Immunization Against Dangerous Childhood Diseases," Southland Corporation in cooperation with the Virginia State Department of Health.
4. "Immunize immunizations," *Virginian-Pilot*, Nov. 27, 1981.
5. Earl Ubell, "How Vaccines May End Infections Forever," *Parade*, Feb. 12, 1984.
6. James Grant, "Simple, Available and Effective Interventions," *A Shift in the Wind*, 18, May 1984, p. 7.
7. "Pioneering doctor predicts 1 vaccine for several diseases," *Virginian-Pilot*, Nov. 9, 1983.
8. "Unborn Children Can Be Immunized Via the Mother," *Washington Post*, Sept. 14, 1983.
9. "Scientists hail new chickenpox vaccine," *Virginian-Pilot*, May 31, 1984.
10. Donna and Stephen Kudabeck, "Opposing Compulsory Immunizations," *Health Freedom News*, April 1984, p. 21.

11. Ibid.
12. The Humanitarian Society, *The Dangers of Immunization*, The Humanitarian Society, Quakertown, Pa., 1979, p. 41. Statement refers to a law passed in England in 1867.
13. Lisa Hogberg, "No shots, no school," *Virginia Beach Beacon*, Aug. 28, 1983.
14. Interview with Clinton Miller, "Vaccination Concerns," *Spotlight*, June 4, 1984.

2

■

ARE IMMUNIZATIONS
HARMLESS?

*Civilization means, above all, an unwillingness to inflict
unnecessary pain. Within the ambit of that definition,
those of us who heedlessly accept the commands of
authority cannot yet claim to be civilized men.*

HAROLD J. LASKI, QUOTED IN STANLEY MILGRAM
Obedience to Authority

FOUR CORNERSTONES

"The judge said that I must present evidence before the next hearing
that vaccinations are harmful or he would have to order shots for Isaac,"
my daughter, Tanya, told me. He told her to turn in the evidence to
the prosecuting attorney at least two weeks before the date of the next
hearing. We turned in almost 90 pages of scientific evidence and opinion
attesting to the harmfulness of vaccinations. Much of the material in
this chapter is taken from that body of evidence and opinion. Since
Tanya was taken to court in 1981 for refusing to have her son vaccinated,
much new material has surfaced. I have included as much of this material
as possible.

Briefly, the four cornerstones upon which the practice of vaccination rests are: (1) Vaccinations are relatively harmless. (2) Vacci-

nations are effective. (3) Vaccinations were primarily responsible for the decline in infectious diseases. (4) Vaccinations are the only practical and dependable way to prevent both epidemics and potentially dangerous diseases.

Let's examine each of these premises (in this and the next two chapters). Later we will examine their implications as well as the mindset that makes each of these assumptions not only possible but an almost inevitable way of perceiving and interpreting certain data.

VACCINES IN GENERAL

The theory of vaccination states that by giving a person a mild form of a disease via the use of immunizing agents, specific antibodies are produced that will protect the organism when the real thing comes along. "This sounds simple and plausible enough except that it doesn't quite work that way," Dr. Alec Burton reminds us.[1] For instance, vaccines, of themselves, as we shall discover, produce a variety of illnesses some of which may be considerably more serious than the disease for which they were given. These vaccine induced diseases may involve "deeper structures, more vital organs, and [have] less of a tendency to resolve spontaneously. Even more worrisome is the fact that they are almost always more difficult to recognize," Richard Moskowitz, M.D., points out.[2]

Besides introducing foreign proteins, and even live viruses into the bloodstream, each vaccine has its own preservative, neutralizer, and carrying agent, none of which are indigenous to the body. For instance, triple antigen DPT (diphtheria, pertussis, and tetanus) contains the following poisons: formaldehyde, mercury (thimersol), and aluminum phosphate (Physician's Desk Reference, 1980). The packet insert accompanying the vaccine (Lederle) lists these poisons: aluminum potassium sulfate, a mercury derivative (thimersol), and sodium phosphate. The packet insert for the polio vaccine (Lederle) lists monkey kidney cell culture, lactalbumin hydrolysate, antibiotics, and calf serum. The packet insert (Merck Sharp & Dohme) for the MMR (measles, mumps, and rubella) vaccine lists chick embryo and neomycin, which is a mixture of antibiotics. Chick embryo, monkey kidney cells, and calf serum are foreign proteins, biological substances composed of animal cells, which, because they enter directly into the bloodstream can become part of our genetic material.[3] These foreign proteins as well as the other carriers and reaction products of a vaccine are potential allergens and can produce anaphylactic shock. "Any person who dies within 15 minutes to a day after taking the vaccine could be suffering from a personal sensitivity, an allergy to the vaccine which is unrelated to the 'dead' viruses therein, most researchers concede."[4] This statement was made in reference to the swine flu vaccine; however, the principle applies to all vaccines.

Another problem with vaccines is that they go directly into the bloodstream without "censoring by the liver," Dr. William Albrecht tells us. "If you take water into your system as drink, it goes into your bloodstream directly from the stomach. But if you take fats, they move into your lymphatic system. When you take other substances like carbohydrates and proteins, they go into the intestines, and from there are passed through the liver, as the body's chemical censor, before they go into the blood and the circulation throughout the body. Most of your vaccination serums are proteins, and are not censored by the liver. Consequently vaccinations can be a terrific shock to the system."[5]

Injections of foreign substances—viruses, toxins, and foreign proteins—into the bloodstream, i.e., vaccinations, have been associated with diseases and disorders of the blood, brain, nervous system, and skin. Rare diseases such as atypical measles and monkey fever as well as such well-known disorders as premature aging and allergies have been associated with vaccinations. Also linked to immunizations are such well-known diseases as cancer, leukemia, paralysis, multiple sclerosis, arthritis, and SIDS (Sudden Infant Death Syndrome).[6] Let's look at the packet inserts of some of the more common vaccines.

MMR AND POLIO VACCINES

From the packet inserts accompanying the polio and MMR (measles, mumps, rubella) vaccines, we learn that paralytic diseases are associated with polio vaccine and that "significant central nervous system reactions such as encephalitis and encephalopathy" can occur after injection with measles, mumps, and rubella vaccine. Reports of ocular palsies, Guillain-Barre syndrome, and subacute sclerosing panencephalitis have occurred after measles vaccination. These are admittedly rare reactions, but some of the more common reactions, which can be "expected to follow administration of monovalent vaccines given separately," are "malaise, sore throat, headache, fever, and rash; mild local reactions such as erythema, induration, tenderness and regional lymphadenopathy; parotitis, orchitis, thrombocytopenia, thrombocytopenia and purpura; allergic reactions such as wheal and flare at the injection site or urticaria; and arthritis, arthralgia and polyneuritis." From Dr. Mendelsohn we learn that measles vaccine can cause "neurologic and sometimes fatal conditions such as ataxia (discoordination), retardation, hyperactivity, aseptic meningitis, seizures, and hemiparesis (paralysis of one side of the body)."[7] Dr. Gregory White says that rubella vaccine can cause rheumatoid arthritis and does not use it in his practice.[8] According to an article in *Science*, in early 1970 the HEW reported that "as much as 26 percent of children receiving rubella vaccination in national testing programs developed arthralgia and arthritis. Many had to seek medical attention, and some were hospitalized to test for rheumatic fever and rheumatoid arthritis."[9]

The Center for Disease Control reports the following side effects of mumps vaccination: Parotitis (inflammation of the parotid glands); allergic reactions, including rash, pruritus and purpura; central nervous system involvement such as fever, seizures, unilateral nerve deafness, and encephalitis within thirty days of mumps vaccination.[10]

In short and in plain language, the MMR and polio vaccines can produce the following pathologies: brain damage; paralysis; nerve inflammation; disease of the lymph glands; inflammation of the testicles and glands near the ear; partial deafness; skin disorders—rashes, tenderness, hardness, itchiness and discoloration; blood disorders; allergies; arthritis.

DPT VACCINE

From the packet insert for the DPT (diphtheria, pertussis, tetanus) vaccine we learn that "symptomology related to neurological disorders" and "excessive screaming syndrome" can follow administration of pertussis antigen. From the Physician's Desk Reference (1980, page 1866) we learn that DPT can cause "fever over 103°, convulsions . . . alterations of consciousness; focal neurologic signs, screaming episodes . . . shock; collapse; thrombocytopenic purpura." Under Side Effects and Adverse Reactions are listed: "1. Severe temperature elevations − 105° or higher. 2. Collapse with rapid recovery. 3. Collapse followed by prolonged prostration and shock-like state. 4. Screaming episodes. . . 5. Isolated convulsions with or without fever. 6. Frank encephalopathy [brain damage] with changes in the level of consciousness, focal neurological signs, and convulsions with or without permanent neurological and/or mental deficit. 7. Thrombocytopenic purpura [blood and skin disorder]. The occurrence of sudden infant death syndrome [SIDS] has been reported following administration of DPT."

"The whooping cough vaccine (a component of the triple antigen

DPT) has such a high percentage of neurologic complications, including death. (sic) Several physicians I know (myself included) do not give it at all," Dr. Mendelsohn tells us.[11] "Dr. Edward B. Shaw, a distinguished University of California physician, has stated (JAMA March 1975): 'I doubt that the decrease in pertussis (whooping cough) is due to the vaccine which is a very poor antigen and an extremely dangerous one, with many very serious complications.' "[12]

Some researchers from Australia have pointed to other serious problems with pertussis vaccine. Drs. Dettman, Kalokerinos, and Ford have pointed to evidence linking pertussis vaccine with the later appearance of asthma and hayfever.[13] Dr. John Fox, of the University School of Medicine, has warned that the risk of paralytic complications may occur with vaccines against measles, polio, whooping cough, and tetanus.[14]

"Many children have suffered horrible and permanent side effects from this vaccine," investigative reporter, Lea Thompson, said on the *Today* show (April 20, 1982). She was referring to the DPT shots given to children, but particularly to the pertussis (whooping cough) component. This 20-minute segment on the *Today* show featuring Ms. Thompson was excerpted from the hour-long documentary "DPT: Vaccine Roulette" which I later saw. This documentary featured children who had been permanently brain damaged as a result of DPT shots. The pictures were pathetic: twisted, uncontrollable bodies, anguished parents, and medical bureaucrats—with three exceptions—repeating the official lines: "The benefits of the vaccine, in my view, far outweigh the risks" and "Much more is to be gained by immunizing the children with the current vaccines with its limitations, than by allowing our children to be exposed to contracting Pertussis."[15]

Some interesting statistics emerged; however, these figures are very conservative because doctors don't report reactions, and what does get reported is the result of some special study commissioned by the government. A recent study at UCLA estimates that as many as one in every 13 children had persistent high-pitched crying after the DPT shot. "This may be indicative of brain damage in the recipient child," Dr. Bobbie Young said. Later on he said, "You know, we start off with healthy infants, and we pop 'em not once, but three or four times with a vaccine . . . the probability of causing damage is the same each time. My greatest fear is that very few of them escape some kind of neurological damage out of this."

One child in 700 has convulsions or goes into shock. "These reactions sometimes cause learning disabilities or brain damage," Ms. Thompson said. These figures represent only the reported effects oc-

curring within 48 hours after the administration of the vaccine. Since
no follow-up studies were done on children after this period, and many
doctors are reluctant to admit that there is a causal relationship between
the administration of the vaccine and later neurological disorders—
probably because of malpractice suits, as well as not wanting to "be
wrong"—the side effects of this vaccine are very underreported.

An even more recent figure on the reaction to the DPT vaccine
indicates that 1 in 100 children react with convulsions or collapse or
high-pitched screaming. One out of 3 of these—that is, 1 in 300—will
remain permanently damaged. According to the testimony of the Assistant Secretary of Health, Edward Brandt, Jr., M.D., before the U.S.
Senate Committee on May 3, 1985, every year 35,000 children suffer
neurological reactions because of this vaccine.[16]

Perhaps the most disturbing statement that most seriously damages
the case for compulsory immunization comes from the above mentioned
DPT documentary. In an interview, F.D.A. official Dr. John Robbins
states: "I think if you as a parent brought your child to a doctor for a
DPT shot and the doctor said to you initially, 'Well, I have to tell you
that some children who get this vaccine get brain damaged,' there's no
question as to what your reaction would be. As a responsible parent
you would say, 'I wish not to take this vaccine.' "

We hear a lot today about hyperactivity and learning disabilities
among children. Who would have imagined that these disorders could
be linked to childhood immunizations? Yet there are doctors and studies
which suggest such a link.[17] Recently I read that one out of eight infants
born in the United States will grow up with some form of mental retardation![18] Could mass immunization programs have something to do
with this grim statistic?

LONG-TERM EFFECTS

This brings us to perhaps the most serious charge against vaccination—
the subtle, long-term effects. Evidence suggests that immunizations
damage the immune system itself. By focusing exclusively on increased
antibody production—which is only one aspect, and by no means the
most important one—of the immune process, immunizations isolate
this function and allow it to substitute for the entire immune response.
Because vaccines "trick" the body so that it will no longer initiate a
generalized inflammatory response, they accomplish what the entire
immune system seems to have evolved to prevent. They place the virus
directly into the blood and give it access to the major immune organs

and tissues without any obvious way of getting rid of it. These attenuated viruses and virus elements persist in the blood for a long time, perhaps permanently. This in turn implies a systematic weakening of the ability to mount an effective response not only to childhood diseases but to other acute infections as well. According to Dr. Richard Moskowitz and others, childhood diseases are decisive experiences in the physiologic maturation of the immune system which prepares the child to respond promptly and effectively to any infections he may acquire in the future. The ability to mount a vigorous, acute response to infectious organisms is a fundamental requirement of health and well-being.[19]

The long-term persistence of viruses and other foreign proteins within the cells of the immune system has been implicated in a number of chronic and degenerative diseases. In 1976, Dr. Robert Simpson of Rutgers University addressed science writers at a seminar of the American Cancer Society and pointed out that

> Immunization programs against flu, measles, mumps, polio and so forth, may actually be seeding humans with RNA to form latent proviruses in cells throughout the body. These latent proviruses could be molecules in search of diseases, including rheumatoid arthritis, multiple sclerosis, systemic lupus erythematosus, Parkinson's disease, and perhaps cancer.[20]

Dr. Wendell D. Winters, a UCLA virologist, communicated similar findings at the same seminar.[21] "Immunization may cause changes in the slow viruses, changes in the DNA mechanism, as being studied by Dr. Robert Hutchinson at the University of Tennessee in Nashville.[22]

Live viruses, the primary antigenic material of vaccines, are capable of surviving or remaining latent within the host cells for years without provoking acute disease. They attach their own genetic material as an extra particle or "episome" to the genome (half set of chromosomes and their genes) of the host cell and replicate along with it. This allows the host cell to continue its own normal functions for the most part, but imposes on it additional instructions for the synthesis of viral proteins. This presence of antigenic material within the host cell cannot fail to provoke autoimmune phenomena such as herpes, shingles, warts, tumors—both benign and malignant—and diseases of the central nervous system such as various forms of paralysis and inflammation of the brain.[23]

If the components of the immune system were designed to help the organism discriminate "self" from "non-self" as a number of researchers believe, then latent viruses, autoimmune phenomena, and cancer would seem to represent different aspects of chronic immune failure, wherein the immune system cannot recognize its own cells as unambiguously its own or eliminate parasites as unequivocally foreign. By the same token, we might say that the inability of the immune system to distinguish between harmful and harmless substances in the environment, as in the case of allergies, constitutes another aspect of chronic immune failure.

Other researchers point to the relationship of immunizations to thymus gland damage and suggest that this might be part of the explanation for the present increase in degenerative diseases.

The immune system produces two functionally distinct kinds of lymphocytes (white blood cells): (1) the B cells which mature largely in the bone marrow and produce antibodies for the control of bacterial infections, and (2) the T cells which originate in the bone marrow but mature in the thymus gland. The T cells protect us from intracellular disorders such as "cancer, virus infections, foreign grafts or transplants, tuberculosis, and various intracellular infections.

"According to sophisticated research . . . at the Arthur Research Corporation, Tucson, Arizona and other centers . . . the effects of childhood vaccine programs on the T-lymphocytes . . . indicate that the immune system becomes 'Substantially committed' after the routine series of vaccines. In other words, a substantial portion of immune bodies (T-lymphocytes) becomes committed to the specific antigens involved in the vaccines. Having become committed, these lymphocytes become immunologically inert, incapable of reacting or defending against other antigens, infections, or diseases. These findings would tend to indicate that the immunological reserve is substantially reduced in many children subjected to standard vaccine programs."[24]

The thymic hormone, *thymosin*, produced by the medullary epithelial cells within the thymus gland, is necessary for the maturation, differentiation, and function of T-lymphocytes throughout the body. Abnormalities in the secretory role of the thymus in production of thymosin are associated with a wide variety of immuno-deficiency, autoimmune and neoplastic diseases. For example, patients with various types of cancers, leukemias, lupus erythematosus, and rheumatoid arthritis usually show impairment of their thymus-dependent immune systems.

Recent investigations in which postmortem examinations were carried out on thymus glands from adult natives in India and Peru showed that the thymus gland did not atrophy in the adult natives, at least not to the extent usually found and reported in the United States. It has long been considered a normal or natural process for the thymus gland to go into rapid atrophy following puberty. The suggestion has been made that the atrophy of the thymus gland found in most adults in the United States is the result of massive vaccination programs.

When the thymus gland is removed from experimental animals there is an increased incidence of tumor formation following exposure of animals to chemical carcinogens and tumor viruses as well as a shortened latency period of tumor development. "Spontaneous cancer development in old age may also be related to declining thymus function and immune responses in old age, at least in those instances in which the cancer cells contain foreign antigens."[25]

The well-known author, lecturer, and health activist, Betty Lee Morales, writes that her parents, who were naturopathic doctors, predicted 50 years ago that cancer would be epidemic in her lifetime as a delayed result of mass vaccinations.[26] Dr. Robert Mendelsohn extends this idea when he says, "I think that most of the degenerative diseases are going to be shown to be due to x-rays, drugs, and polluted food, additives, preservatives and immunizations."[27]

"With all our discoveries about the effects on the human body of ingesting substances not found in nature, one thing we ought to know by now is that many of these toxins—and vaccinations are toxins by definition—kill slowly or kill only after the lapse of significant periods of time," Nicholas von Hoffman said in his *Washington Post* column.[28]

MORE CASUALTIES

Two Australian doctors, Drs. Glen Dettman and Archie Kalokerinos, felt so strongly about the destructive effects of vaccines that in 1976 they engaged in a worldwide campaign to warn people against all vaccines: "Vaccines are killing children. There's no doubt about it. We've got figures to show it. It's damaging them, and in the United Kingdom there is now a society for parents of vaccine-damaged children," they said in an interview with Jay Patrick.[29]

The *British Medical Journal* (Feb. 1976) published the following letter from Rosemary Fox, Secretary, Association of Parents of Vaccine-Damaged Children:

"Two years ago, we started to collect details from parents of serious reactions suffered by their children to immunizations of all kinds. In 65 percent of the cases referred to us, reactions followed 'triple' vaccinations. The children in this group total 182 to date; all are severely brain damaged, some are also paralyzed, and 5 have died during the past 18 months. Approximately 60 percent of reactions (major convulsions, intense screaming, collapse, etc.) occurred within 3 days and all within 12 days."[30]

One of the leading bacteriologists of our time, and Professor of Bacteriology at the London School of Hygiene and Tropical Medicine, Sir Graham S. Wilson, M.D., L.L.D.,F.R.C.P.,D.P.H., wrote in his book, *The Hazards of Immunization*:

> The risk attendant on the use of vaccines and sera are not as well recognized as they should be . . . The late Dr. J. R. Hutchinson, of the Ministry of Health, collected records of fatal immunological accidents during the war years, and was kind enough to show them to me. I was frankly surprised when I saw them to learn of the large number of persons in the civil and military population that had died apparently as the result of attempted immunization against some disease or other. Yet, only a very few of these were referred to in medical journals . . . And further, when one considers that such accidents have probably been going on for the last 60 or 70 years, one realizes what a very small proportion have been described in the medical literature of the world.[31]

From West Germany we read of more vaccination casualties. A reader writing to *Organic Consumer Report* (June 13, 1968) mentions an article which appeared in *Medical World* which stated that about 3,000 children each year suffer varying degrees of brain damage as the result of smallpox vaccination. This same writer mentions another medical journal in which Dr. G. Kittel, M.D., reported that in the previous year, smallpox vaccination damaged the hearing of 3,296 children in West Germany and 71 became totally deaf. Hearing loss was reported by Dr. William Albrecht who said in the article quoted earlier in this chapter, that a typhoid shot he received made him stone deaf in one ear as well as deathly ill at the time of the shot.

Thus far our discussion has revolved around numbers and nomenclature, making it too easy to forget that these abstractions represent people, real human tragedies. So, to flesh out our discussion, let us look briefly at a few case histories compiled by Lily Loat, for many years secretary of the National Anti-Vaccination League of Great Britain.

Dennis Hillier, a healthy English boy who excelled in running, swimming, football, and other games, died in October 1942 of a rare form of encephalitis, some two months after his second inoculation. He had reacted to an initial inoculation with slightly confused speech, but no one had connected this reaction with the inoculation. In describing the case, Dr. W. Russell Brain said at a meeting of the Section of

Neurology of the Royal Society of Medicine in February 1943, "The patient, a boy of eleven, developed symptoms after anti-diphtheria inoculation." After mentioning several other cases of nervous disorders and poliomyelitis occurring within a few days after inoculation against diphtheria, he added, "the relation of the infection to the inoculation was at present unsettled."

Christine Timms, a 13-month-old English child who had not been ill since birth, died in February 1949, five days after she had been inoculated against diphtheria. The pathologist said the death was due to septicaemia due to septic tonsillitis.

A five-year-old child, Sylvia Harrison Laplage, died in July 1949, a few days after inoculation against diphtheria. The death certificate gave the cause of death as "Toxaemia of unknown origin."[32]

It goes on, case after case. Rarely is the cause of death ever listed as vaccinia. Asthma, acute lymphatic leukaemia, streptococcal cellulitis, tubercular meningitis, and infantile paralysis are some of the causes of death listed on the death certificate.

More graphic descriptions of children dying—frequently after terrible suffering—from the effects of vaccination can be found in Eleanor McBean's book, *The Poisoned Needle*. Many of the cases have accompanying photographs of the children showing gaping wounds, festering sores, sightless eyes and withered limbs as the result of vaccination. By the side of a picture of a beautiful baby girl we read:

> Margaret Ann, the only daughter of Mr. and Mrs. Donald W. Gooding, of Wolsey, Essex, England, was pronounced a perfect baby by the doctor when she was born. This beautiful and healthy infant was vaccinated at the age of 4 months. The first two injections didn't take so a third was given, after which inflammation of the brain developed within 5 days. She was taken to the hospital where she remained for many weeks. At the age of 13 months she was blind and could not learn to walk. She also developed digestive disturbances and convulsions.[33]

Interviews with over 100 parents of vaccine damaged children and stories of the subsequent medical coverups are reported in the recently published *DPT: A Shot in the Dark*, by Harris L. Coulter and Barbara Loe Fisher. A few of the interviews are published in detail; all are heartbreaking—beautiful, healthy babies killed or damaged for life. One mother, for example, whose son died 33 hours after his first DPT shot, confronted her pediatrician and was met with denials, even though she pointed out to him that her first son had the same reaction after his shot. The coroner also tried to deny any connection, writing on the death certificate "death due to irreversible shock." even after the mother explained in detail what had happened. "He said he couldn't write down on the death certificate that Richie had died from a DPT reaction because 'the state's standing on immunizations would be in an uproar.' "[34]

A couple of years ago I read a case of a girl turned into a "vegetable" (post vaccinal encephalitis) from a smallpox vaccination (*Washington Post*, September 9, 1981). I remembered Jack Ashley, a member of the British Parliament, saying that vaccination has turned some children into "cabbages." "Over a 25-year period, 300 children in Britain had been deafened, blinded, or suffered permanent brain damage after immunization against whooping cough, diphtheria and tetanus. Happy healthy children have been turned into cabbages within a few days."[35] "Dozens of children die each year, and thousands are severely harmed and crippled for life, as a direct result of vaccinations," Dr. Airola tells us.[36] Is it any wonder that some doctors have called vaccinations "legalized child abuse"?[37]

At this point one might ask, "How does such a destructive practice manage to survive for so long?" The answer is simple: The equation, "Disease prevention equals vaccination" and its corollary "Mass immunization programs equal prevention of epidemics" are writ large in the public mind. I won't go into the complexities of who is responsible for this public image except to suggest that those who make money from this practice—namely the medical/pharmaceutical industry—appear to be implicated.

NOTES

1. Alec Burton, O.D., "The Fallacy of the Germ Theory of Disease," talk given at the convention of the National Hygiene Society, Milwaukee, Wis., 1978.
2. Richard Moskowitz, M.D., *The Case Against Immunizations*, reprinted from the *Journal of the American Institute of Homeopathy*, vol. 76, March 1983, p. 10.
3. *World Medicine*, Sept. 22, 1971, pp. 69–72; *New Medical Journals Limited*, Clareville House, pp. 26–27, Oxendon St., London, J. W. 1X4 EL, England. Reprinted in part in *The Dangers of Immunization*, published by the Humanitarian Publishing Company, Quakertown, Pennsylvania, 1979, pp. 20–31.

4. Jay Patrick, "The Great American Deception," *Let's Live*, Dec. 1976, p. 58.
5. *Organic Consumer Report*, Dec. 4, 1962.
6. *Physician's Desk Reference*, 1980, p. 1866. *Organic Consumer Report*, April 19, 1977; Organic Consumer Report, April 29, 1969. Also the works of Drs. Mendelsohn, Moskowitz, Airola, Dettman, Kalokerinos and others, many of whose works are referred to in this and other chapters.
7. Robert Mendelsohn, M.D., *Confessions of a Medical Heretic*, Contemporary Books, Chicago, 1979, pp. 142–45.
8. Robert Mendelsohn, M.D., *The People's Doctor*, "Immunization Update," Vol. 4, No. 5, p. 8.
9. *Science*, March 26, 1977, reported by Donna Benson, "Vaccine Aftermath," *Health Freedom News*, July/Aug. 1984, p. 29.
10. Mendelsohn, *People's Doctor*, p. 4.
11. Robert Mendelsohn, M.D., "Vaccinations Pose Hazards, Too," *Idaho Statesman*, Dec. 19, 1977.
12. *Journal of the American Medical Association*, March 10, 1975, p. 1026.
13. Drs. Kalokerinos and Dettman, "A Supportive Submission," *The Dangers of Immunisation*, Biological Research Institute, Warburton, Victoria, Australia, 1979, p. 74.
14. Drs. Archie Kalokerinos and Glen Dettman, " 'Mumps' the word but you have yet another vaccine deficiency," *The Australasian Nurses Journal*, June 1981, p. 17.
15. Drs. Edward Mortimer (American Academy of Pediatrics) and John Robbins (FDA, Bureau of Biologics) respectively.
16. Betty Kamen, Ph.D., "A Shot in the Dark," *Health Freedom News*, May 1985, p. 38.
17. P. Landrigan and J. Witte, "Neurologic Disorders Following Live Measles Virus Vaccination," 223 *Journal of the American Medical Association*, 1459, March 26, 1973. Also, Harris L. Coulter and Barbara Loe Fisher, *DPT: A Shot in the Dark*, Harcourt Brace Jovanovich, New York, 1985, Chapters 7 and 8.
18. "Book Shelf," *Better Nutrition*, June 1982, 32. (Review of the book, *Growing Better Babies*, by Daniel Elam, Ph. D.)
19. Moskowitz, op. cit., p. 14.
20. Ibid. page 23.
21. Betty Lee Morales, "What's Your Problem?", *Let's Live*, Dec. 1976.
22. Robert Mendelsohn, M.D., "More Confessions," Interview, *The Herbalist New Health*, July 1981, p. 60.

23. Moskowitz, op. cit., p. 15.
24. Drs. Kalokerinos and Dettman, "A Supportive Submission," *The Dangers Of Immunisation*, Biological Research Institute, Warburton, Victoria Australia, 1979, p. 49.
25. Ibid., pp. 51–53.
26. Morales, op. cit.
27. Robert Mendelsohn, M.D., Interview, *Public Scrutiny*, March 1981, p. 22.
28. Nicholas von Hoffman, "Free Immunity Shots: Pros and Cons," *Washington Post*, Nov. 28, 1977.
29. Patrick, op. cit., p. 57.
30. Paavo Airola, *Everywoman's Book*, Health Plus Publishers, P.O. Box 22001, Phoenix, Ariz. 85028, 1979, p. 281.
31. Ibid., p. 284.
32. Lily Loat, *The Truth About Vaccination and Immunization*, Health for All Publishing Co., London, 1951, pp. 53 - 55.
33. Eleanora McBean, *The Poisoned Needle*, Health Research, Mokelumne Hill, Calif., (undated), p. 78.
34. Harris L. Coulter and Barbara Loe Fisher, *DPT: A Shot in the Dark*, Harcourt Brace Jovanovich, New York, 1985, p. 10.
35. *Organic Consumer Report*, "Cabbage Heads—London, England," (from a reader's letter), April 19, 1977.
36. Paavo Airola, N.D., Ph.D., "Nutrition Forum," *Let's Live*, Dec. 1976.
37. Drs. Dettman and Kalokerinos, "Immunizations—What Are Your Rights?" *Toorak Times*, Oct. 11, 1981, Victoria, Australia.

3

■

ARE IMMUNIZATIONS
EFFECTIVE?
(THE STATISTICAL MILL)

Ignorance is not not knowing but knowing what isn't so.

MARK TWAIN

THE DECLINE
OF INFECTIOUS DISEASES

Do vaccines protect us from the diseases for which they are given? This question might seem absurd on the face of it, given the near disappearance of many infectious diseases for which vaccines are given credit. A closer look, however, at the effectiveness of vaccines, as well as a look at some of the methods of gathering and interpreting statistical data, reveals some interesting discrepancies.

Are vaccinations primarily responsible for the decline of infectious diseases? Actual statistics and records form around the world show that infectious diseases, e.g., smallpox, diphtheria, whooping cough, scarlet fever, etc., began to disappear long before immunizations ever came on the scene.[1] According to the *World Health Statistics Annual, 1973–1976*, Volume 2, there has been a steady decline of infectious diseases "in most 'developing' countries regardless of the percentage of immunizations administered in these countries. It appears that generally improved conditions of sanitation are largely responsible for preventing 'infectious' diseases."[2]

What about the decline in tuberculosis, chicken pox, scarlet fever, typhus, typhoid and the plague for which there are no routine immunizations? A number of researchers including the distinguished biologist, Rene Dubos, have pointed out that infectious diseases disappeared as the result of sanitation and public water supplies. Other researchers have included improved personal hygiene and better distribution and increased consumption of fresh fruits and vegetables.[3] When Jonathan Miller, M.D., was interviewed on the Dick Cavett show (Feb. 4, 1981), he pointed to improved ventilation and drainage, along with nutrition, as being the primary determinants responsible for the decline in the death rate. (He also said that in the past 50 years modern medicine has made such an insignificant contribution to human health and longevity that the enormous expense incurred was hardly worth it.)

An article with the droll title, "'Mumps' the word but you have yet another vaccine deficiency," appeared in the *Australasian Nurses Journal* (June, 1981) in which Dr. Glen Dettman and Dr. Archie Kalokerinos discuss not only the new mumps vaccine being promoted but the efficacy of all vaccines. Besides pointing out that 90 percent of the so called "killer diseases" had all but disappeared when immunizations were introduced on a large scale (see figure 1, page 25), they say that "since the introduction of routine immunisations we now have an ever alarming increase of degenerative diseases and maladies, but worse still, the diseases we are supposed to be protected from still occur, probably in larger numbers than we might have expected them to, had we simply allowed the declining disease rate as exemplified by the graph to continue." The doctors also point to an editorial that appeared in the *Lancet* (Dec. 1, 1980) which tells that the BCG vaccine (tuberculosis vaccine) was a failure and that there was a greater incidence of tuberculosis in the vaccinated. In another article these same doctors mention that in their own country of Australia where tuberculosis vaccinations were given, some of the strain of bacteria mutated, killing around 600 children.[4]

The recitation of statistics that pro-vaccinationists love to use to "prove" the effectiveness of mass immunization programs are classic examples of *post hoc* reasoning, the fallacy of "after therefore because of" (post hoc ergo propter hoc). "Permitting statistical treatment and

Figure 1 below was presented at the Presidential Address of the British Association for the Advancement of Sciences (Porter, 1971), and Figure 2 appeared in an article published in Scientific American, written by Professor John Dingle (1973). These two countries are widely separated, but the conclusions are similar.

THE IMMUNIZATION MYTH?

England & Wales: Deaths of children under 15 years attributed to scarlet fever, diphtheria, whooping cough and measles (Porter, 1971).

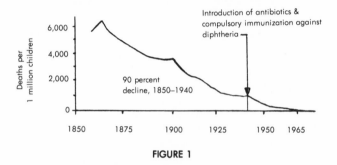

FIGURE 1

THE IMMUNIZATION MYTH?

Declining death rates attributable to infectious diseases of infancy and child-hood, such as tuberculosis (upper curve) and typhoid fever (lower curve). No immunization against TB has been adopted in the U.S. The effectiveness of typhoid vaccine is questionable (Dingle, 1973).

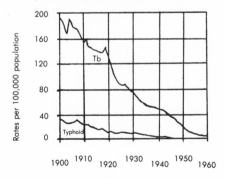

FIGURE 2

The Dangers of Immunisation, The Humanitarian Society, Quakertown, Pa., enlarged and republished by the Biological Research Institute, Warburton, Victoria, Australia.

the hypnotic presence of numbers and decimal points to befog causal relationships is little better than superstition," Darrell Huff tells us in his delightful little book, *How to Lie With Statistics*. After pointing out some humorous examples of positive correlations of unrelated events made to appear as though they were causally related, he says that "scantier evidence than this—treated in the statistical mill until common sense could no longer penetrate it—has made many a medical fortune and many a medical article in magazines, including professional ones."[5]

Before a causal relationship can be established between any two events the following criteria must be satisfied: (1) Controls. Was there a control group? What were the controls used? (2) Variables. What were the variables? Were they controlled? (3) Size and duration. Were the number of participants and the duration of the experiment adequate? In other words, when a causal relationship is implied, we must ask ourselves, "What other factors are involved and what are the controls?"

Polio

Let's look at the statistical mill itself. The case of poliomyelitis is particularly instructive since its apparent decrease cannot be explained by such developments as sanitation, public water supplies, ventilation, etc. In fact, it is a disease that occurs only among the most civilized peoples with the highest standards of sanitation, etc., being unknown among preliterate cultures that have been relatively untouched by civilization.

Jonas Salk, the discoverer of the Salk polio vaccine, has been called the "twentieth-century miraclemaker" and the savior of countless lives.[6] We read glowing reports of the dramatic decrease in poliomyelitis in the United States as a result of the Salk vaccine. For instance, the Virginia State Department of Health distributes a folder which tells us that polio vaccines have reduced the incidence of polio in the United States from 18,000 cases of paralytic polio in 1954 to fewer that 20 in 1973–78. A recent article in *Modern Maturity* states that in 1953, there were 15,600 cases of paralytic polio in the United States; by 1957, due to the Salk vaccine, the number had dropped to 2,499.[7]

During the 1962 Congressional Hearings on HR 10541, Dr. Bernard Greenberg, head of the Department of Biostatistics of the University of North Carolina School of Public Health, testified that not only did polio increase substantially (50 percent from 1957 to 1958 and 80 percent from 1958 to 1959) *after* the introduction of mass and frequently compulsory immunization programs, but statistics were manipulated and statements made by the Public Health Service to give the opposite impression.[8]

For instance, in 1957 a spokesman for the North Carolina Health Department made glowing claims for the efficacy of the Salk vaccine, showing how polio steadily decreased from 1953 to 1957. His figures were challenged by Dr. Fred Klenner who pointed out that it wasn't until 1955 that a single person in the state received a polio vaccine injection. Even then injections were administered on a very limited basis because of the number of polio cases resulting from the vaccine. It wasn't until 1956 "that polio vaccinations assumed 'inspiring' proportions." The 61 percent drop in polio cases in 1954 was credited to the Salk vaccine when it wasn't even in the state! By 1957 polio was on the increase.[9]

Other ways polio statistics were manipulated to give the impression of the effectiveness of the Salk vaccine were: (1) Redefinition of an epidemic: More cases were required to refer to polio as epidemic after the introduction of the Salk vaccine (from 20 per 100,000 to 35 per 100,000 per year). (2) Redefinition of the disease: In order to qualify for classification as paralytic poliomyelitis, the patient had to exhibit paralytic symptoms for at least 60 days after the onset of the disease. Prior to 1954 the patient had to exhibit paralytic symptoms for only 24 hours! Laboratory confirmation and the presence of residual paralysis were not required. After 1954 residual paralysis was determined 10 to 20 days and again 50 to 70 days after the onset of the disease. Dr. Greenberg said that "this change in definition meant that in 1955 we started reporting a new disease, namely, paralytic poliomyelitis with a longer lasting paralysis." (3) Mislabeling: After the introduction of the Salk Vaccine, "Cocksackie virus and aseptic meningitis have been distinguished from paralytic poliomyelitis," explained Dr. Greenberg. "Prior to 1954 large numbers of these cases undoubtedly were mislabeled as paralytic polio."[10]

Another way of reducing the incidence of disease by way of semantics—or statistical artifact, as Dr. Greenberg calls it—is simply to reclassify the disease. From the Los Angeles County Health Index: Morbidity and Mortality, Reportable Diseases, we read the following:

Date	Viral or Aseptic Meningitis	Polio
July 1955	50	273
July 1961	161	65
July 1963	151	31
Sept. 1966	256	5

7

The reason for this remarkable change is stated in this same publication: "Most cases reported prior to July 1, 1958, as non-paralytic poliomyelitis are now reported as viral or aseptic meningitis."[11] In *Organic Consumer Report* (March 11, 1975) we read, "In a California Report of Communicable Diseases, polio showed a 0 count, while an accompanying asterisk explained, "All such cases now reported as meningitis."

There have been at least three major polio epidemics in the United States, according to Dr. Christopher Kent. "One occurred in the teens, another in the late thirties, and the most recent in the fifties." The first two epidemics simply went away like the old epidemics of plague. Around 1948, the incidence of polio began to soar. (Interestingly, this is when pertussis—whooping cough—vaccine appeared, Dr. Kent points out.) It reached a high in 1949, with 43,000 cases, but by 1951 had dropped to below 28,000. In 1952, when a government subsidized study of polio vaccine began, the rate soared to an all-time high of well over 55,000 cases. After the study, the number of cases dropped again and continued to decline as they had in the previous epidemics. "This time, however, the vaccine took the credit instead of nature."[12]

The cyclical nature of polio is again illustrated by the remarks of Dr. Alec Burton at the 1978 meeting of the Natural Hygiene Society in Milwaukee, Wisconsin. Some years ago at the University of New South Wales in Australia, statistics were compiled which showed that the polio vaccine in use at the time had no influence whatsoever on the polio epidemic. Polio comes in cycles anyway, Dr. Burton said, and when it has been "conquered" by vaccines, and a disease with identical symptoms continues to appear, doctors look for a new virus because they know the old one has been "wiped out." "And the game goes on," he added.[13]

When Dr. Robert Mendelsohn was asked about the possibility of childhood diseases—particularly polio—returning if the vaccinations were stopped, he replied: "Doctors admit that forty percent of our population is not immunized against polio. So where is polio? Diseases are like fashions; they come and go, like the flu epidemic of 1918."[14]

On a 1983 Donahue Show ("Dangers of Childhood Immunizations," Jan. 12), Dr. Mendelsohn pointed out that polio disappeared in Europe during the 1940s and 1950s without mass vaccination, and that polio does not occur in the Third World where only 10 percent of the people have been vaccinated against polio or anything else.

Returning to the congressional hearings referred to earlier (HR 10541), we read that in 1958 Israel had a major "type I" polio epidemic *after* mass vaccinations. There was no difference in protection between the vaccinated and the unvaccinated. In 1961, Massachusetts had a "type III" polio outbreak and "there were more paralytic cases in the triple vaccinates than in the unvaccinated."[15]

Testimony at these same hearings from Herbert Ratner, M.D., pointed out that because poliomyelitis is such a low-incidence disease, this complicates the evaluation of a vaccine for it. He also said that there is "a high degree of acquired immunity and many natural factors preventing the occurrence of the disease . . . in the Nation at large."[16]

Dr. Moskowitz adds that the virulence of the poliovirus was low to begin with. "Given the fact that the poliovirus was ubiquitous before the vaccine was introduced, and could be found routinely in samples of city sewage whenever it was looked for, it is evident that effective, natural immunity to poliovirus was already as close to being universal as it can ever be, and *a fortiori* no artificial substitute could ever equal or even approximate that result."[17]

MMR and DPT

What about the rest of the standard repertoire of vaccines for children in the United States—measles, mumps, rubella, diphtheria, whooping cough, and tetanus? Since we have concerned ourselves so far with large numbers and population studies, let's look briefly at a few small-scale studies.

"The World Health Organization did a study and found that while in an unimmunized, measles-susceptible group of children the normal rate of contraction of disease was 2.4 percent; in the control group that had been immunized, the rate of contraction rose to 33.5 percent."[18] On a 1983 Donahue Show ("Dangers of Childhood Immunizations," Jan.12), Dr. J. Anthony Morris pointed out that in a recent measles epidemic in Dade County, Florida, most of the cases occurred in vaccinated children.

Let's look again at the statistical mill with regard to measles. From 1958 to 1966, the number of measles cases reported each year dropped from 800,000 to 200,000. The drug industry claims this drop was due to vaccinations; however, there are some interesting discrepancies: (1) The incidence of measles has been declining steadily for the past 100 years. (2) It wasn't until 1967 that the live vaccine which is presently used was introduced because the killed virus vaccine which came out in 1963 was found to be ineffective and potentially harmful. (3) A survey of pediatricians in New York City revealed that only 3.2 percent of them were actually reporting measles cases to the health department. (4) In 1974, the Centers for Disease Control determined that there were

36 cases of measles in Georgia, but the Georgia state surveillance system reported 660 cases that same year.[19]

The statistical mill is worth looking at with respect to whooping cough "epidemics." Because physicians have a stake in vaccination programs, "there is a natural tendency to underreport whooping cough when it occurs in a vaccinated population, and to overreport it when it appears to be occurring in an unvaccinated population," Coulter and Fisher report (*DPT: A Shot in the Dark*). When vaccination rates decline, physicians tend to diagnose pertussis "every time a baby clears his throat," Dr. Mendelsohn tells us. Within a few months after "DPT: Vaccine Roulette," was aired (April 1982), the states of Maryland and Wisconsin reported whooping cough "epidemics." The Maryland state health officials implied that this rise in cases was the result of parents seeing the documentary and not having their children vaccinated. The cases in both the Maryland and Wisconsin "epidemics" were analyzed by J. Anthony Morris, Ph.D., an expert on bacterial and viral diseases. In Maryland, he found laboratory confirmation in only five out of the 41 cases and all of them had been vaccinated! In Wisconsin, he found laboratory confirmation in only 16 out of 43 cases, and all but two had been vaccinated![20] The formula seems to be: If you want to sell vaccines—and visits to the doctor—create epidemics.

The effectiveness of whooping cough vaccine has been reported to be about 50 percent. Of 8,092 cases of whooping cough reported in the British Medical Journal, 36 percent were immunized and 30 percent unimmunized.[21] Hardly 50 percent protection.

What about rubella? Dr. Plotkin, Professor of Pediatrics at the University of Pennsylvania School of Medicine states, "It is clear that vaccination of children (for rubella), which has only been done for several years, is not very successful as a policy." Thirty-six percent of adolescent females who had been vaccinated against rubella lacked evidence of immunity by blood test, he points out. In another study reported by the University of Minnesota a high serological (pertaining to serums) failure rate was shown in children given rubella, measles, and mumps vaccine.

A large proportion of children are found to be seronegative (no evidence of immunity in blood tests) four to five years after rubella vaccination.[22] In another study, 80 percent of army recruits who had been immunized against rubella came down with the disease. The same results were shown in a consecutive study that took place at an institution for the mentally retarded.[23]

"Cook County, Ill., hospital decided to immunize one-half of the nursing staff and not the other half. Diphtheria broke out soon afterward among the immunized cases, not the others. It invaded both halves, both the immunized and the unimmunized, and the total of cases was much higher among the supposedly immunized cases than among those not immunized."[24]

"During a 1969 outbreak of diphtheria in Chicago, four of the sixteen victims had been 'fully immunized against the disease,' according to the Chicago Board of Health. Five others had received one or more doses of the vaccine, and two of these people had tested at full immunity. In another report of diphtheria cases, three of which were fatal, one person who died and fourteen out of twenty-three carriers had been fully immunized."[25]

Sometimes diphtheria has increased to epidemic proportions *after* the introduction of mass compulsory vaccination. For instance, diphtheria increased by 30 percent in France, 55 percent in Hungary and tripled in Geneva, Switzerland *after* the introduction of mass compulsory immunization. "In Germany, where compulsory mass immunization was introduced in 1940, the number of cases increased from 40,000 per year to 250,000 by 1945, virtually all among immunized children." "On the other hand, in Sweden, diphtheria virtually disappeared without any immunizations."[26] "In major U.S. epidemics during the past decade, the diphtheria immunization had failed to demonstrate effectiveness in terms of cases or deaths."[27]

Could the real reason vaccination promise and performance seem so contradictory is that the vaccination premise itself is faulty? As stated earlier, the theory of vaccination postulates that the use of immunizing agents produces a mild form of a disease for which specific antibodies are formed that will protect the body when the real thing comes along. As we saw, it doesn't quite work that way. Dr. Alec Burton points out, for instance, that there are children with agamma globulin anemia, which means that they are incapable of producing antibodies, yet these children develop and recover from measles and other zymotic (infectious or contagious) diseases almost as spontaneously as other children.

He describes an interesting study in England that was carried out in 1949–50 and published by the British Medical Council in May 1950 in their report #272. The study investigated the relation of the incidence of diphtheria to the presence of antibodies. Since diphtheria was epidemic at or just prior to the time of the study, the researchers had a large number of cases to investigate. The purpose of the research was to determine the existence or non-existence of antibodies in people who developed diphtheria and those who did not but were in close proximity to those who did, such as physicians, nurses working in hospitals, family, and friends. The conclusion was that there was no relation whatsoever between the antibody count and the incidence of disease. The researchers found people who were highly resistant with extremely low antibody counts, and people who developed the disease who had high antibody counts. The study was finally abandoned because of the extremely conflicting data.[28]

The mystery begins to unravel when we look at the work of Drs. Dettman and Kalokerinos. In one of their articles they quote Dr. Wendel Belfield of San Jose, California, who says, "Antibodies are not needed when the primary immunological defense (leukocytes, interferon etc.) is functioning at maximum capacity. . . . Antibody production appears to occur only when the ascorbate level, in the primary defense components are at low levels thereby permitting some viruses to survive the primary defense."[29]

Smallpox

No discussion of immunization would be complete without including smallpox since the World Health Organization (WHO) is now claiming that their global smallpox immunization campaign has rid the world of smallpox. One dissenter, Professor Arie Zuckerman, who is a member of the World Health Organization's advisory panel on viruses, warned against the smallpox vaccine saying, "Immunization against smallpox is more hazardous than the disease itself." We now have "monkeypox" which, according to the weekly epidemiological record of WHO (54:12–13, 1979), is clinically indistinguishable from smallpox.[30]

The chicanery sometimes used in compiling vaccination statistics is discussed in much of the literature distributed by The National Anti-Vaccination League in Britain. For instance, "the Ministry of Health itself has admitted that the vaccinal condition is a guiding factor in diagnosis."[31] This means that if a person who is vaccinated comes down with the disease he is "protected" against, the disease is simply recorded under another name; for example, "in the thirty years ending in 1934, 3,112 people are stated to have died of chicken-pox, and only 579 of smallpox in England and Wales. Yet all authorities are agreed that chicken-pox is a non fatal disease."[32] In other words, people who have been vaccinated for smallpox and later come down with the disease are classified in the health records as having chickenpox. "This has been admitted by English medical officers of health, and the Ministry of Health has twice stated in answer to questions in Parliament that vaccination is one factor in the diagnosis of these cases."[33]

George Bernard Shaw said, "During the last considerable epidemic at the turn of the century, I was a member of the Health Committee of London Borough Council, and I learned how the credit of vaccination is kept up statistically by diagnosing all the revaccinated cases (of smallpox) as pustular eczema, varioloid or what not—except smallpox."[34]

The cycles of mandatory vaccinations for smallpox and the terrible smallpox epidemics that followed would take many pages to chronicle, so let's just look at a few samples: "For more than fifty years the populations of Australia and New Zealand (with the exception of the armed forces in time of war) have been practically unvaccinated, and they have been more free from smallpox than any other community." "The most thoroughly vaccinated countries are Italy, the Philippine Islands, Mexico and what was formerly called British India. And all of these have been scourged with smallpox epidemics."[35]

"Our U.S. Government staged a compulsory vaccination campaign in the Philippines which brought on the largest smallpox epidemic in the history of that country with 162,503 cases and 71,453 deaths, all vaccinated. That was between 1917 and 1919."[36]

In England the "ghastly epidemic of 1871–1872 broke out after 13 years of voluntary inoculations, followed by 18 years of a mandatory program, backed up by four years of Draconian [very severe] punishments" for those refusing vaccinations, writes Fernand Delarue in his book, L'intoxication Vaccinale. At the time of the epidemic's outbreak, 90 percent of the population was believed to have been vaccinated.[37]

"Japan started compulsory vaccination against smallpox in 1872 and continued it for about 100 years with disastrous results. Smallpox increased every year. By 1892 their records showed 165,774 cases with 29,979 deaths, all vaccinated. In Australia where they had no compulsory vaccination they had only 3 deaths from smallpox in 15 years."[38]

But the answer to the riddle of smallpox—and polio—is found in the next chapter.

FROM ACUTE TO CHRONIC DISEASE

As we have seen, statistical argument can be deceptive, so let's suppose that disease can be prevented by artificial immunization. (This is the practice of injecting toxic substances into the body as opposed to natural immunization that occurs as the result of natural infection and/or certain living habits which we shall discuss later.) There is, however, a very disturbing question we should ask ourselves: Could artificial immunization suppress disease symptoms arising from imbalances—for example, biochemical deficiencies and toxicity—and drive the disease deeper into the body where it might later manifest in more dangerous and disabling ways? I am reminded of what William Howard Hay, M.D., said in this connection:

> "And if you have been dealing as I have with the derelicts from all over the world for 30 years, you would find an almost fatal relationship between this history of vaccination and some failing that follows this for many years that has kept a person from being as well as he should have been.[39]

Richard Moskowitz, M.D., states the case more specifically:

> "It is dangerously misleading, and, indeed, the exact opposite of the truth to claim that a vaccine makes us "immune" or *protects* us against an acute disease, if in fact it only drives the disease deeper into the interior and causes us to harbor it *chronically*, with the result that our responses to it become progressively weaker, and show less and less tendency to heal or resolve themselves spontaneously.[40]

Vaccines have been called potential allergins because they introduce foreign proteins directly into the blood without digestion or "censoring by the liver." When we remember that one of the chief causes of allergies is the presence of undigested proteins in the blood, the connection between immunizations and allergies becomes apparent. In Chapter 8 we shall discuss in more detail how immunizations along with other drugs route acute illnesses into their chronic form.

Perhaps a fairly straightforward illustration of how vaccines can work to suppress rather than prevent disease can be found in the example of measles. Although outbreaks of measles continue to occur among supposedly immune school children, the peak incidence of measles now occurs in adolescents and young adults where the risk of pneumonia and demonstrable liver abnormalities has increased substantially to well over 3 percent and 2 percent respectively.

The syndrome of "atypical measles"—pneumonia, petechiae (skin blotching), edema, and severe pain—is not only difficult to diagnose but is often overlooked entirely. Likewise, symptoms of atypical mumps—anorexia, vomiting, and erythematous (red) rashes, without any parotid (near the ear) involvement—require extensive serological testing to rule out other concurrent diseases.

As with measles, outbreaks of mumps and rubella among supposedly immune school children continue to be reported. Again, however, both these diseases which are essentially benign, self-limited diseases of childhood, are being transformed by a vaccine into considerably less benign diseases of adolescents and young adults. In the case of mumps, the chief complication is epididymoorchitis (acute inflammation of the testicles) which occurs in 30 to 40 percent of males affected after the age of puberty. This usually results in atrophy of the affected testicle. Mumps can also "attack" the ovary and pancreas.

When rubella occurs in older children and adults it not only can produce arthritis (as can the vaccine), purpura (skin discoloration), and other severe systemic disorders but "congenital rubella syndrome" (damage to the developing embryo during the first trimester of pregnancy), the very disease the vaccine was designed to prevent in the first place.[41]

ARTIFICIAL
VERSUS NATURAL IMMUNITY

When immunity to a disease is acquired naturally, the possibility of reinfection is only 3.2 percent, journalist Marian Tompson tells us. If the immunity comes from a vaccination, the chance of reinfection is 80 percent.[42] In one study of military recruits, the reinfection rate was 80 percent compared with 4 percent in naturally immune individuals.[43]

Dr. William Howard Hay has pointed out that in any epidemic of communicable disease only a small percentage of the population contracts the disease. Most people are naturally immune; so if a man who has been vaccinated does not contract the disease that really proves nothing. If he had not been vaccinated the chances are he would not have contracted the disease anyway. We have no way of knowing. In a sense we have destroyed our evidence.[44]

"Just because you give somebody a vaccine, and maybe get an antibody reaction, doesn't mean a thing. The only true antibodies, of course, are those you get naturally," Dr. Dettman said in an interview with Jay Patrick. "What we're doing is interfering with a very delicate mechanism that does its own thing. If nutrition is correct, it does it in the right way. Now if you insult a person in this way and try to trigger off something that nature looks after, you're asking for all sorts of trouble, and we don't believe it works."[45]

"Natural diseases are a lot safer than acute artificial complications," Dr. Mendelsohn reminds us.[46]

Perhaps the strongest statement against the effectiveness of artificial immunization comes from Dr. William Howard Hay. "It is nonsense to think that you can inject pus . . . into a little child and in any way improve its health. . . . There is no such thing as immunization, but we sell it under the name—immunization. . . . If we could by any means build up a natural resistance to disease through these artificial means, I would applaud it to the echo, but we can't do it. The body has its own methods of defense. These depend on the vitality of the body at the time. If it is vital enough, it will resist all infections; if it isn't vital enough it won't and you can't change the vitality of the body for the better by introducing poison of any kind into it."[47]

Notes

1. Robert Mendelsohn, M.D., talk at the National Health Federation Conference in Orlando, Fla., Feb. 1980. Other researchers who have pointed out the same thing include: Paavo Airola, N.D., Ph.D., *Everywoman's Book*, Health Plus, Phoenix, Ariz., 1979, p. 274; Rene Dubos, *Mirage of Health*, Anchor Books, Garden City, New York, 1961, pp. 30, 70, 31, 129, 130; *The Dangers of Immunization*, Harold Buttram, M.D., The Humanitarian Society, Quakertown, Pa., 1979, pp. 48–56; Drs. Dettman and Kalokerinos, M.D.'s, "'Mumps' the word but you have yet another vaccine deficiency," *The Australasian Nurses Journal*, June 1981. Also the same doctors interviewed by Jay Patrick, "The Great American Deception," *Let's Live*, Dec. 1976, p. 57.
2. Leonard Jacobs, "Menage," *East/West Journal*, Sept. 1977, p. 15. The World Health Statistics Annual is published by the World Health Organization, Geneva, Switzerland.
3. Mendelsohn, Airola, Dubos, Buttram, Drs. Dettman and Kalokerinos, op. cit. Also, an interesting study by W. J. McCormick, M.D., "The Changing Incidence and Mortality of Infectious Disease in Relation to Changed Trends in Nutrition," *Medical Record*, Sept. 1947, credits the increased consumption of vitamin C rich foods, particularly citrus and tomatoes, as well as improved nutrition and hygiene with the decline of infectious diseases.
4. Dettman and Kalokerinos interviewed by Jay Patrick, "The Great American Deception," *Let's Live*, Dec. 1976, p. 57.
5. Darrell Huff, *How to Lie with Statistics*, W.W. Norton, New York, 1954, Chapter 8.
6. Joan S. Wixen, "Twentieth-century miraclemaker," *Modern Maturity*, Dec. 1984–Jan. 1985, p. 92.
7. Ibid.
8. Hearings before the Committee on Interstate and Foreign Commerce, House of Representatives, Eighty-Seventh Congress, Second Session on H.R. 10541, May 1962, p. 94

9. "The Disturbing Question of the Salk Vaccine," *Prevention*, Sept. 1959, p. 52
10. Hearings on H.R. 10541, op. cit., pp. 94, 96, 112.
11. Christopher Kent, D.C., Ph.D., "Drugs, Bugs, and Shots in the Dark," *Health Freedom News*, Jan. 1983, p. 26.
12. Ibid.
13. Alec Burton, O.D., "The Fallacy of the Germ Theory of Disease," talk given at the convention of the National Hygiene Society, Milwaukee, Wis., 1978.
14. Interview with Robert Mendelsohn, M.D., *The Herbalist New Health*, July 1981, p. 61.
15. Hearings on 10541, op. cit., p. 113.
16. Ibid. pp. 89, 94.
17. Richard Moskowitz, M.D., *The Case Against Immunizations*, reprinted from the *Journal of the American Institute of Homeopathy*, vol. 76, March 1983, p. 21.
18. Paavo Airola, N.D., Ph.D., *Everywoman's Book*, Health Plus, Phoenix, Ariz., 1979, p. 279.
19. Marian Tompson, "Another View," *The People's Doctor*, Vol. 6, No. 12, p. 8.
20. Harris L. Coulter and Barbara Loe Fisher, *DPT: A Shot in Dark*, Harcourt Brace Jovanovich, New York, 1985, pp. 164–68.
21. Airola, op. cit., p. 272
22. Robert Mendelsohn, M.D., *The People's Doctor*, "Immunization Report II", Vol.4, No. 5, p. 3.
23. Airola, op. cit., p. 276.
24. William Howard Hay, M.D., quoted by Usher Burdick in the House of Representatives, 1937. (Congressional Record, Dec. 21, 1937.)
25. Robert Mendelsohn, M.D., *Confessions of a Medical Heretic*, Contemporary Books, Chicago, 1979, p. 143.
26. Airola, op., cit., p. 277.
27. Mendelsohn, *The People's Doctor*, pp. 1, 5.
28. Burton, op. cit., talk given in 1978.
29. Drs. Glen Dettman and Archie Kalokerinos, Ph. D. and M.D. respectively, "A Supportive Submission," *The Dangers of Immunization*, published and written by the Humanitarian Society, Quakertown, Pa., 1979. Australian edition published by the Biological Research Institute, Warburton, Victoria, Australia, pp. 79–80.
30. Ibid. p. 75.
31. M. Beddow Bayly, *The Case Against Vaccination*, Wm H. Taylor & Sons, Ltd., Printers, York Road, London, June 1936, p.4.
32. Ibid. p. 5.
33. Lily Loat, address given before the English Annual Session of the

American Medical Liberty League, reprinted by *The Truth Teller*, "Philosophy of Health," Jan. 1927.

34. Eleanora McBean, *The Poisoned Needle*, Health Research, Mokelumne Hill, Calif. (undated), p. 64.
35. Lily Loat, *The Truth About Vaccination and Immunization*, Health for All Publishing Company, London, 1951, p. 28.
36. Harold Buttram, M.D., *The Dangers of Immunization*, The Humanitarian Society, Quakertown, Pa., 1979, p. 48.
37. Ibid. p. 47.
38. Ibid. p. 48.
39. Hay, op. cit., 1937.
40. Moskowitz, op. cit., p. 13.
41. Ibid. pp. 9–10. Also Tompson, op. cit.
42. Tompson, op. cit.
43. Mendelsohn, *The People's Doctor*, op. cit., p. 3.
44. Hay, op. cit., The actual percentage of persons (prior to 1937) affected by the epidemics for which we now have vaccinations are: (1) Not more than 10 percent of the general population and (2) Not more than 15 percent of the childhood population in the case of diphtheria.
45. Patrick, op. cit., p. 57.
46. Alice Karas, Interview with Robert Mendelsohn, M.D., "More Confessions," *Herbalist New Health*, July 1981, p. 60.
47. Hay, op. cit., 1937.

4

∎

CREATING NATURAL IMMUNITY

Follow principle and the knot unties itself.

THOMAS JEFFERSON

FIRST PRINCIPLES

If we can't prevent disease by injecting toxins into our bodies, how can we prevent it? First of all, we must begin by thinking health, rather than disease; of building or creating something desirable, rather than avoiding or destroying something undesirable. Freedom from illness is a by-product of thinking and building health, not of fighting disease. Essentially, we build health by positive thinking and balanced living. This latter includes biochemical balance which is supported by eating fresh, whole, natural foods that have not been refined, chemicalized, and overcooked. Both herbs and megadoses of vitamin C have been used successfully to either prevent infectious diseases or to shorten their duration and lessen their discomfort.[1]

Currently the focus is on megadoses of vitamin C to protect people from bacterial assaults. Other researchers prefer to think of vitamin C

as helping to correct body chemistry. It is this latter interpretation that
we will follow, partly because it is more constructive to think of disease
as something we build from within rather than something that attacks
us from without. Also, research that we will later explore supports this
more endogenous—and, I think, more holistic—point of view.

THREE BOOKS

In 1939, 1949, and 1951 three books were published that support this
more endogenous theory of disease. They have made a major contribution to our understanding of how both infectious and degenerative
diseases are built from within by our habits of living and thinking. Few
people have heard of these books because they are "dangerous." If the
ideas they contain were widely disseminated, they would topple much
of the present medical-pharmaceutical establishment. The first and most
dangerous book is *The Chemistry of Natural Immunity*, written by a
man who was not only a doctor of medicine but a doctor of biochemistry
as well. The author, Dr. William Frederick Koch, discusses his research
and presents case histories from his own medical practice. He discovered
that homeopathic doses of oxidation catalysts injected at cyclical inter-
vals along with a regimen of "fresh pure air, pure water, plenty of rest,
and reasonable exercise" and a diet of whole, natural foods—"vegetable, fruit and whole grain cereal diet, avoiding coffee, tea, chocolate,
alcohol, spices, tobacco"—and "the use of bowel lavage with salt water
when necessary" would support the oxidation mechanism of the body
and facilitate natural immunity to disease.*

The case histories in the book are impressive: Cancer, poliomyelitis,
psoriasis, epilepsy, arthritis, allergies, toxic goitre, etc., respond to this
therapy, most with complete recoveries.[2]

The Koch treatment, as it is called, is of particular significance to
me because of a personal experience I had with it. About 18 years ago
while living in California, I had a severe attack of asthma as a result of
an unusually stressful experience.** I went to a medical doctor who
specialized in using nutritional and other "natural" therapies, and he

---

*We can think of the oxidation process as cell respiration. When this process is blocked,
disease results.

**As a child I had hayfever for which I was treated by the usual "shots." This eventually
resulted in asthma which became incapacitating and which I corrected by changing my
diet to one of "natural" foods—whole grains, raw milk, fresh fruits and vegetables, fertile
eggs, and occasionally fresh fish, fowl, and organ meats. Because this treatment was not
"holistic"—meaning the mind and emotions were not addressed—a sufficiently stressful
experience could trigger an "episode" of asthma.

gave me an injection of what he said was an early form of the Koch oxidation catalysts (developed by Dr. Koch in the early years of his practice). Within a few hours after receiving the injection, I experienced a distinct feeling of euphoria and well-being. I found myself breathing deeply and having several loose bowel movements a day as though my body were discharging toxins. My asthma disappeared and has never returned. The immediacy and apparent permanence of my response was no doubt due, at least in part, to the fact that I was already living on a program very much like the one Dr. Koch recommended. Because the Koch treatment is illegal in this country, the doctor who treated me had to send to Switzerland for the Koch catalyst. The Koch catalysts are not toxic or dangerous physiologically, only dangerous politically and economically.

Our second book, *Diet Prevents Polio*, by Benjamin Sandler, M.D., tells how a polio epidemic in Asheville, North Carolina, was averted when the author got on the radio and warned parents not to feed their children sugar and foods containing sugar—soft drinks, ice cream, candy, and the like—and to reduce consumption of fruits and fruit juices. Dr. Sandler recommended a high protein diet with low starch vegetables as being the best protection against low blood sugar, a condition he found made people susceptible to polio. Polio epidemics occur during the summer, he said, because this is the time people consume high sugar foods as well as fruits and fruit juices. (Later researchers have vindicated fruit and fruit juices provided they are unsweetened with refined sugar. They say, in effect, that because the sugar in these natural foods is in a different form and is accompanied by other food factors it is metabolized in a different way than are refined sugars.) The typical polio "profile," Dr. Sandler found, is heavy physical exertion coupled with high consumption of refined carbohydrates—refined flour and sugar products, particularly sugar.

That the Sandler diet does prevent polio is illustrated not only by Dr. Sandler's research with rabbits and monkeys, but also by case studies on human beings and the remarkable reduction of polio in North Carolina after the Sandler diet was publicized on the radio and in the newspapers. The incidence of polio in North Carolina dropped from 2,402 cases in 1948 to 214 cases in 1949 when the country as a whole— 39 states—showed an increase in the number of cases from 1948 to 1949![3] One of the reasons polio has declined in the U.S. is the decreased consumption of refined sugar, due in part to the increased consumption of alternative sweeteners.*

*Although we are consuming record quantities of sweeteners—133 pounds per person in 1984—much of this consists of alternative sweeteners such as honey, maple syrup, fruit

Another researcher, J. W. McCormick, M.D., of Toronto, Canada, has pointed out that the first case of poliomyelitis was reported in Vienna one year after roller-mill white flour was first sold there. Dr. McCormick calls polio the form of beri-beri that follows the use of degerminated flour.[4]

Other researchers have linked polio to DDT poisoning, pointing out that American servicemen in the Philippines and elsewhere in the Far East who used "vast quantities of DDT as insecticides, had a high incidence of polio, whereas it was extremely low in the surrounding native population." Other researchers have indicted other poisons which affect the nervous system.[5] Still others have indicted the high intake of white sugar and sugar products as being a primary cause of polio among U.S. servicemen stationed overseas, particularly when the native population with whom the soldiers mingled freely were free of disease.[6]

Our third book, *Bacteria, Inc.*, tells the story of the discovery of the cause, prevention, and cure of smallpox. The author, Cash Asher, describes the research of the distinguished medical doctor, Charles A. R. Campbell, who was recommended for the Nobel Prize around the turn of the century. Dr. Campbell made notable contributions in researching typhoid and malaria as well as smallpox. He discovered that smallpox, like malaria, was carried by a blood-sucking insect, that the disease was neither infectious nor contagious, and that vaccinations do not prevent it. Although Drs. Campbell and Watts, and others, disclosed their findings at the turn of the century, their reports were ignored.

Through a series of carefully controlled experiments, Dr. Campbell discovered that smallpox was caused by the bite of *cimex lectularius*, a Latin name for bedbug. (Around the turn of the century bedbugs were a common household pest. Straw-filled mattresses and straw padded rag carpets, the natural breeding place of the bedbug, were standard household furnishings.) Dr. Campbell also discovered that the degree of severity of the disease was directly proportional to the *cachexia* (general ill-health and malnutrition) of the patient. He spoke of "scorbutic cachexia," relating it to scurvy, "the disease caused by lack of green food," and said that "the removal of this perversion of nutrition will so mitigate the virulence of this malady as positively to prevent the pitting or pocking of smallpox."[7] In other words, eating lots of fresh greens

concentrates, and chemical sweeteners. Refined sugar consumption in 1984 was 67.5 pounds per person compared to 89.2 in 1975 (*East West*, May 1986, p. 36). According to the latest Statistical Abstract (107th), we consumed 63 pounds of sugar per person in 1985. This is 35 pounds less than we consumed in 1960 and 38 pounds less than in 1950. These statistics, however, don't include the sugar in processed, packaged foods such as ice cream, pop, ketchup, etc. With the increased public awareness of the deleterious effects of sugar, there is, no doubt, a marked decrease in overall sugar consumption.

will prevent the scarring of smallpox. My guess is that eating a balanced diet of whole, fresh foods including fresh greens, will prevent not only the scarring of smallpox but will lessen the discomfort and duration of the disease as it does for other diseases.

If this sounds a bit simplistic, given the enormous mystique surrounding smallpox and its prominent place in history, one need only look to 18th-century England to discover that the consumption of fresh fruits and vegetables was a rarity, particularly among the poorer classes who ate mostly cereal foods. An English country gentleman's dinner in 1768 would include: "A roasted Shoulder of Mutton and a plum Pudding—Veal Cutlets, Frill'd Potatoes, cold Tongue, Ham and cold roast Beef, and eggs in their shells. Punch, Wine, Beer and Cyder for drinking."[8]

Smallpox, along with typhus (caused by body lice), plague (caused by lice on rats), typhoid and cholera (caused by contaminated water) have been called "filth" diseases. When we read about the great epidemics that swept through Europe and England hundreds of years ago killing up to three-fourths of the population, as did the black plague in the 14th century, it is hard for us to imagine the living conditions which spawned them:

"No sewers, no water closets, but instead, festering privies; excessive over-crowding, both of houses per acre and people per house; small, ill-ventilated and ill-built houses crammed into narrow courts and tortuous alleys, without adequate water supply and devoid of sanitary conveniences; lack of cleanliness owing to scarcity of water; absence of baths and laundry facilities; unpaved and ill-paved streets, which were made the receptacle for all kinds of slops and other filth. . . .

"In addition to constantly breathing in the horrible effluvia from the stinking heaps of rotting refuse and filth from vaults containing sewage heaps and from their own unwashed clothes and bedclothes, the poor suffered badly in periods of scarcity and want. . . .

"In the seventeenth and eighteenth centuries bad harvests were almost always followed by a large increase in the number of deaths from smallpox and fevers.[9]

"History shows that famine and pestilence commonly ride together," Rene Dubos tells us. "Susceptibility to infection . . . appears to be linked in a reversible manner to the metabolic state."[10] Again, we find the importance of diet in building health and reducing susceptibility to disease.

Changing patterns of living produce changing patterns of disease: As straw-filled mattresses and straw-padded rag carpets were discarded along with fly-infested privies, mosquito-infested rain barrels, and food cooled in cellars rather than in refrigerators, smallpox, along with other "dirt" diseases, disappeared. Likewise, tetanus, which is caused by a spore found in horse manure and fecal matter in general, has practically disappeared with the advent of the "horseless carriage" and the flush toilet. And now in our sanitized world we have degenerative diseases such as heart trouble, cancer, arthritis, multiple sclerosis, polio, and hyperkinesis. These are due, at least in part, to our consumption of refined carbohydrates, devitalized and chemicalized food, exposure to agricultural and industrial poisons, and yes, immunizations.

COVERUP

What happened to the information contained in the three books discussed above? Why isn't this information general knowledge? In the words of Cash Asher: "Why, then, does the vaccination fetish persist? We must find the answer in economics—in the billion dollar serum industry and its correlative industry, medical practice."[11] In the television documentary, "Pesticides and Pills," which aired on Public Television in the latter part of 1981, Dr. Milton Silverman, A University of California pharmacologist, said that the pharmaceutical industry "is now grossing sales in the tens of billions of dollars a year." Any business that controls such large sums of money becomes an irresistible political and economic force which puts its stamp on legislation and subsequently education. When the bedbug was exposed as the carrier of smallpox, the manufacturing of serums had grown into a profitable industry. Many states and cities had enacted laws and regulations making vaccination compulsory, and the vaccination of every child before entering school had become an established practice. Doctors were finding vaccinations a lucrative part of their practice. Is it any wonder that Dr. Campbell's attempts to communicate his discoveries were ignored?

In the case of polio and Dr. Sandler, I heard in a public lecture many years ago that hundreds of thousands of dollars worth of soft drinks, ice cream, and candy went unsold, precipitating heavy losses for the businesses involved. Referring to Asheville, North Carolina, Dr. Sandler said, "Store sales of sugar, candy, ice cream, cakes, soft drinks, and the like dropped sharply and remained at low level for the rest of the summer. One southern producer of ice cream shipped one million fewer gallons of ice cream than usual, during the first week following the release of the diet story."[12] Like Dr. Campbell, Dr. Sandler's work was ignored by public health officials and the medical community in general. I suspect pressure from big business—which includes medical-pharmaceutical "big business"—kept the story under wraps.

The discoveries of Dr. Koch met with much more drastic action. His therapy was too revolutionary and too threatening to the medical-pharmaceutical business to be merely ignored or hushed up. He was actively persecuted and prosecuted, much as doctors are today who use laetrile or other metabolic therapies. Many years ago I read about arrests, trials, defamation, heartache, and eventual "escape" to Brazil where Dr. Koch spent his later years helping the Brazilian government eliminate diseases of cattle and other livestock.

THE BEST "VACCINE"

A question frequently asked is, "If natural immunity is so effective, how is it that native peoples such as the North, South, and Central American Indians and the Polynesians frequently experienced such devastating epidemics when they first came into contact with white men?" These people obviously ate "natural foods" and yet when white man brought his western civilization to them they died in large numbers— at least, according to some accounts. The key here is "brought his western civilization to them." This civilization included not only canned, preserved, and refined foods which native people frequently accepted as gifts from the newcomers, but a great deal of negativity as well, as stories of exploitation and cruelty attest. Also, their native diets, even before the advent of white man, were not always balanced, being subject to the vagaries of weather and tribal customs. However, it does appear that as long as they lived on their native foods, they were relatively free from disease. Only when they adopted white man's foods did disease ravage their numbers.

In his book, *Nutrition and Physical Degeneration*, Dr. Weston A. Price documents the results of his trip around the world to many remote areas where native peoples lived relatively untouched by modern civilization. In every case, he found that people who lived on their native diets were not only free from disease but were free from the skeletal deformities that characterized native people who had adopted white man's foods.[13]

Frequently we hear that native people succumbed to white man's diseases because they had no natural immunity, the implication being that either artificial immunization or longer and more gradual exposure would have given them that immunity. It seems, rather, that their departure from their traditional food patterns destroyed their immunity, and that, had they remained on a diet of their traditional foods, they would have retained their immunity.

"Even the World Health Organization has conceded that the best vaccine against common infectious diseases is an adequate diet. Despite this, they made it perfectly clear to us that they still intended to promote mass immunization campaigns," Drs. Kalokerinos and Dettman tell us. "Do we take this as an admission that we cannot or do not wish to provide an adequate diet? More likely it would seem, there is no profit in the constituents of an adequate diet for the pharmaceutical companies."[14]

CHILDREN "IN JEOPARDY"?

"In jeopardy" is a term frequently used by pediatricians to refer to an unvaccinated child. Suppose your child does contract a "dread" disease like whooping cough, diphtheria, polio, etc. What can you do that is simple, harmless, and effective? As I pointed out earlier, megadoses of vitamin C have been known to both shorten the duration of many infectious diseases as well as lessen their discomfort. Used along with herbs, particularly alfalfa, and a non-mucus forming diet,* the vitamin C is rendered more effective. Let's look at a few cases where vitamin C alone was used.

According to the *Journal of the American Medical Association*, Nov. 4, 1950, 90 children with whooping cough were treated daily with 500 mg. of vitamin C, intravenously and orally, for one week. Every second day the dosage was reduced by 100 mg. until it was 100 mg. a day. This last dose was given continually until each child was completely recovered. Children receiving vitamin C intravenously were well in 15 days, those receiving vitamin C orally were well in 20 days. The children treated with vaccine averaged 34 days duration. In three-quarters of the cases when vitamin C therapy was started in the catarrhal stage, the spasmodic stage was wholly prevented.[15]

Adelle Davis used much higher potencies and administered them orally. She describes how her own children weathered most of the childhood diseases with only one day of sickness—no nausea, no vomiting, no irritability, and no missed meals. For her five-year-old son's

---

*A non-mucus forming diet consists primarily of fresh fruits and vegetables, whole grains and legumes, some fish and fowl and no dairy or flour products.

"one-day mumps" she began at 7 A.M. to give him 1,000 mg. of vitamin C every hour during the day. By evening all swelling was gone and there was no further sign of illness. To administer this high a potency orally to a small child it is necessary to dissolve fifty 500 mg. tablets of vitamin C in a cup of boiling water and mix it with one-fourth cup of fruit juice such as pineapple, apricot, or orange. Each teaspoonful of the solution would then contain 500 mg. of vitamin C. Later, Adelle Davis would discover that lesser amounts of vitamin C are needed when calcium and pantothenic acid (vitamin B5) are included in the dosage. (I, personally, have found using the entire C complex—bioflavinoids, rutin, hesperidin—more effective than just the ascorbic acid fraction.)

If the illness seems more serious, larger doses can be taken. Adelle Davis describes again how her sleeping three-year-old daughter had the classical symptoms of illness—elevated temperature, flushed and burning skin, labored breathing. She gave 2,000 mg. of the dissolved vitamin C in juice, and in 15 minutes her temperature was normal. She slept soundly the rest of the night and awoke the next day "full of her usual vivacity."[16] In this case, the remarkable degree of effectiveness of this treatment is due, in large part I think, to the fact that Adelle Davis fed her children an exceptionally healthful diet.

Amounts of vitamin C needed vary greatly according to the usual diet and tissue saturation with the vitamin as well as with the severity of the disease. Dr. Fred Klenner, for instance, describes an 18-month-old girl whose body was blue, stiff, and cold to the touch; he could neither hear her heart nor feel her pulse. The mother was convinced the child was already dead. "Dr. Klenner injected 6,000 mg. of vitamin C into her blood; four hours later the child was cheerful and alert, holding a bottle with her right hand, though her left side was paralyzed. A second injection was given; soon the child was laughing and holding her bottle with both hands, all signs of paralysis gone."[17]

But even without these megadoses of vitamin C, the child who is well nourished can handle these "dread" diseases without much discomfort. My own children, who were never vaccinated, came down with whooping cough, the younger child being only two weeks old! Because I was nursing her, our doctor—a naturopath, chiropractor, and iridologist—said just to keep nursing her and she would be all right. I've forgotten the advice he gave for my older daughter, but the disease was certainly not horrendous in the least. Annoying, inconvenient, and, at times, uncomfortable, but certainly not "dread." Had I known about giving children megadoses of vitamin C, the duration of the disease could have been shortened and the discomfort of the spasmodic stage eliminated. As it was, the disease lasted six weeks including two weeks of the spasmodic stage. Yet I heard on a TV program a few years ago that in England whooping cough could last three and sometimes four months! I am sure a child fed a balanced diet of "natural" foods would not experience the disease that severely. I, along with Dr. Mendelsohn, would rather have the disease than the vaccination.

When we talk about natural foods for infants and small children, we are talking about breast milk, not formula milk. We are also talking about fresh fruits and vegetables, (can be blended in blender), not canned; and whole (preferably germinated) grains, not packaged cereals.

Vitamin C is not necessarily the *sine qua non* of natural or drugless healing. Other natural substances such as herbs have been used successfully in treating—and preventing—"infectious" diseases.[18] Just plain alfalfa—tablets or capsules—have been used successfully to prevent whooping cough as well as to build stronger bodies in children.[19] And, of course, garlic is an old folk remedy for preventing infectious diseases.

Iodine has been used successfully to both prevent and treat various paralytic diseases including polio. Dr. J. F. Edward, M.D., writing in the *Manitoba Medical Review* for June–July 1954, told of his success in treating and preventing polio with potassium iodide. He also listed 25 different references which reported the work of other doctors and veterinarians who had successfully treated and prevented various paralytic diseases, including herpes zoster and encephalitis, with potassium iodide.[20] Later, *Prevention* magazine distributed a flier describing an article Dr. Edward wrote in the *Canadian Medical Journal* (Sept. 1, 1955) in which he showed that not only could iodide be used for treating polio, but suggested that lack of iodine in the diet might be a contributing cause of this disease. *Prevention*'s editors speculate that one reason why polio might be more prevalent in hot weather is that iodine is lost in the perspiration along with other minerals.

Another doctor, DeForest Clinton Jarvis, M.D., found that polio is accompanied by a disturbance in the calcium-potassium and calcium-phosphorous ratio of the blood. He successfully treated polio in both man and animals by using, for the most part, simple, natural treatments designed to raise the blood calcium and lower the blood phosphorous. Some of these are: (1) With each meal, drinking a glass of water to which has been added two teaspoonfuls of honey and two teaspoonfuls of apple cider vinegar; (2) Applying hot moist applications to the affected parts; (3) Drinking certain herb teas; (4) Using a sedative diet, one which eliminates all wheat products, citrus fruits, and muscle meats such as beef, lamb, and pork; (5) Giving injections of insulin as needed; and (6) For adults, using ten drops of a saturated solution of potassium iodine in a glass of water after each meal. Using only kelp, a natural source of iodine, Dr. Jarvis cured a paralyzed chinchilla.[21]

Magnesium has also been used successfully to arrest polio. Dr. A. Neveu of France reported complete reversal of this disease within two days to one week, even after early arm and leg paralysis. Dr. Neveu uses magnesium chloride and claims rapid results are realized when correctly used. His formula: 20 grams (.7 oz) of desiccated magnesium chloride added to one liter (about one quart) of water. The dose varies from 80 cc. every three hours to 125 cc. every six hours. Magnesium should be used under the care of a qualified physician, Dr. Neveu advises.[22]

Like Dr. Edward, the famous medical clairvoyant, Edgar Cayce, recommended iodine as a preventative of polio. He recommended using Atomidine, a solution carrying iodine in atomic form, and he gave instructions for using it both internally and externally as a wash and as a throat and nasal spray.

Also, like a number of doctors mentioned earlier, Edgar Cayce thought more in terms of preventing disease by changing body chemistry rather than by "fighting germs." He said that if the body were maintained in an alkaline condition this would "immunize" a person against infectious diseases. When a young woman asked him, "Can immunizations against them [infectious diseases] be set up in any other manner than by inoculations?" he replied, "As indicated, if an alkalinity is maintained in the system —especially with lettuce, carrots and celery, these in the blood supply will maintain such a condition as to immunize a person." He specified that alkaline vegetables—lettuce, carrots, and celery—must be eaten every day.[23] Keeping the body alkaline, by using predominantly alkaline-forming foods* in the diet as a means of preventing disease, has long been taught by doctors such as Bernard Jensen who use natural therapies. And where does vitamin C fit into this picture? Vitamin C creates an alkaline ash within the body.

SOCIETY "IN JEOPARDY"?

Are unvaccinated persons a danger to others? At this point, the question is rhetorical, and I ask it only because parents who choose not to have

---

*Alkalinity and acidity refer to the final metabolic residue of a food after it is "burned" or digested. To keep our bodies alkaline, 80 percent of our diets should consist of fresh fruits and vegetables. This figure varies somewhat with the age and life-style of the person as well as the season and climate.

their children vaccinated will likely be confronted by people who think their decision a selfish one and their children a public health threat. This happened to my daughter, Tanya, when she refused to have her son immunized. One of the arguments of the prosecuting attorney was that "society has rights."

To a person whose understanding of the nature of bacteria and their relation to disease consists of a world inhabited by unseen enemies who attack unprotected persons, this fear of contamination by the unvaccinated is quite real. However, if they themselves are protected what have they to fear? As Clarence Darrow said, "If vaccination does what its advocates claim for it, the person who is vaccinated ought to be safe no matter whether anybody else is vaccinated or not." "There is no rationale for forcing immunization," said Dr. J. Anthony Morris, former chief vaccine control officer of the FDA, who was fired for blowing the whistle on the swine flu vaccine program.[24]

Do the "unprotected" ever stop to think that there are probably hundreds of thousands of unvaccinated "threats" living among them? Besides an increasing number of families like ours who simply don't buy into the paradigm, there are those who object on religious grounds, for example, Christian Scientists, Church of Life Science in Texas, Lord's Covenant Church in Arizona, and others. No one seems to think that people who refuse vaccination for religious reasons pose a threat to the community. In fact, Dr. Mendelsohn says that the life expectancy records of the Christian Scientists are one of the best in the country.[25]

We are living in an age of alternatives, of energies and images that liberate us from cultural monoliths. We speak of alternative schooling, alternative life styles, alternative health care. We speak of becoming "conscious." To become conscious we must become aware of our viewing lenses and the assumptions that have shaped and colored them. We can't really become aware of our assumptions until we expose ourselves to realities based upon different assumptions.

Let's begin our journey into greater consciousness by going "through the looking glass" and exploring a world that is almost a mirror image of our present world, a world in which the understanding of our relationship to disease, health, and microorganisms is the reverse of our present one, a world in which the villain becomes the hero, the mischief maker the teacher, and the sickness the process by which the body—and society—heals itself.

But first we must turn back the pages of time and find a chapter in the history of biology that was lost.

NOTES

1. Walene James, "Immunization Law Based on Myth," *Health Freedom News*, Oct. 1983.
2. William Frederick Koch, M.D., *The Chemistry of Natural Immunity*, The Christopher Publishing House, Boston, 1939. Quotations are from p. 105.
3. Benjamin P. Sandler, M.D., *Diet Prevents Polio*, The Lee Foundation for Nutritional Research, 1951. Figures are quoted from p. 43.
4. Royal Lee, D.D.S., "Food Integrity—The Foundation of Health," Address to the Organic Health Foundation of America, Jan. 20, 1955.
5. Morton S. Biskind, M.D., "Public Health Aspects of the New Insecticides," The *American Journal of Digestive Diseases*, Nov. 1953, p. 334.
6. Sandler, op. cit., pp. 68–73. Other articles which support this same line of reasoning are: (1) W. J. McCormick, M.D., "Poliomyelitis, Infectious or Metabolic?", *Archives of Pediatrics*, 67:56–73, Feb. 1950. (2) R. H. Scobey, "The Poison Cause of Poliomyelitis and Obstructions to Its Investigation," *Archives of Pediatrics*, 69:172–93, April 1952. (3) R. H. Scobey, "Is the Public Health Law Responsible for the Poliomyelitis Mystery?", ibid., 68:220–32, May 1951.
7. Cash Asher, *Bacteria, Inc.*, Bruce Humphries, Inc., Boston, 1949, pp. 36–7.
8. Henry E. Sigerist, *Civilization and Disease*, Cornell University Press, Ithaca, N. Y., 1943, p. 14.
9. Lily Loat, *The Truth About Vaccination and Immunization*, Health for All Publishing Company, London, 1951, p. 7.
10. Rene Dubos, "Second Thoughts on the Germ Theory," *Scientific American*, May 1955, p. 34.
11. Asher, op. cit., p. 42.
12. Sandler, op. cit., pp. 35–6.
13. Weston A. Price, *Nutrition and Physical Degeneration*, The American Academy of Applied Nutrition, Los Angeles, Calif., 1939.
14. Archie Kalokerinos and Glen Dettman, M.D.s, "A Supportive Submission," *The Dangers of Immunisation*, Biological Research Institute, Warburton, Victoria, Australia, 1979, p. 68. (Originally written by and published by the Humanitarian Society in Quakertown, Pa., and enlarged and republished by the Biological Research Institute, Australia.)

15. J. C. de Wit, abstr., *Journal of the American Medical Association* 144 (Nov. 4, 1950): 879.
16. Adelle Davis, *Let's Eat Right to Keep Fit*, Harcourt, Brace and Company, New York, 1954, pp. 146–47.
17. Ibid., p. 143.
18. John Christopher, *Childhood Diseases*, 1978, Christopher Publications, P.O. Box 412, Springville, Utah 84663, discusses herbal remedies helpful in treating childhood diseases.
19. From a flier distributed by Shaklee supervisor, Irma Ahola, "Alfalfa," John W. Shenton, Johannesburg, South Africa (undated).
20. J. F. Edward, M.D., "Iodine, Its Use in the Treatment and Prevention of Poliomyelitis and Allied Diseases," *Manitoba Medical Review*, June–July 1954, Vol. 34; No. 6:337–39.
21. D. C. Jarvis, M.D., "The Use of Honey in the Prevention of Polio," *American Bee Journal*, Vol. 91, No. 8, Aug. 1951, pp. 336–37.
22. Linda Clark, *Get Well Naturally*, ARC Books, Inc., New York, N.Y., 1972, pp. 120–21.
23. Edgar Cayce, Reading #480-19. Cayce specified in a number of readings that if one would avoid colds and flu he must "keep the body alkaline." The Cayce readings are filed numerically in the library of the Association for Research and Enlightenment at Virginia Beach.
24. Reported by a reader in *Organic Consumer Report*, April 25, 1978.
25. Robert Mendelsohn, M.D., "The Truth About Immunizations," *The People's Doctor*, April 1978, p. 6.

PART II

■

BEYOND DISEASE WARS

Either war is obsolete or men are.

R. BUCKMINSTER FULLER

5

■

DO GERMS CAUSE
DISEASE OR DOES
DISEASE CAUSE GERMS?

Two roads diverged in a wood, and I—
I took the one less traveled by.
And that has made all the difference.

ROBERT FROST, "THE ROAD NOT TAKEN"

A LOST CHAPTER
IN THE HISTORY OF BIOLOGY[1]

Are there forks in the roads of history and choices that make "all the difference"? Is our way of thinking about disease— particularly infectious disease—largely the result of a choice that was made around the middle of the last century? Was this choice the result of a fork in the road in which we took one path and not the other? Is the road we didn't take more salutary, less conducive to commercial exploitation and therefore "the road not taken"?

Let's go back to the scientific world of about 130 years ago. Scientists were arguing about the origin and nature of living matter and were asking such questions as: What is the "thing" that causes milk to sour, meat to spoil, and wine to ferment? Where does it come from?

55

Does it come from the air? Does it grow from other matter? Or does it just appear from nowhere?

Most scientists believed the "thing" (living matter) that caused fermentation appeared from nowhere. This theory was called "spontaneous generation." One French scientist, however, proved through experiments in his laboratory that fermentation was the result of living organisms and that these organisms are airborne. They grow in the food and ferment it by a process of their digestion, assimilation, and excretion.

Does this sound like I am talking about Louis Pasteur? Read on.

This same scientist also discovered that living organisms exist within cells as well as on external surfaces and that these organisms can cause fermentation as can airborne organisms.

Meanwhile, another scientist, a spontepartist (one who believes in the spontaneous generation of matter) seized upon this first scientist's ideas and claimed them as his own. Being extraordinarily ambitious man with a genius for self-promotion, he popularized as well as plagiarized the original scientist's ideas when he found that his own observations and explanations would not stand up to scrutiny. This plagiarism—the first of many such plagiarisms—would not have been so devastating had the ideas not been oversimplified and distorted. For instance, having realized that airborne microorganisms (later known as bacteria) caused fermentation, he became fixated and sought to explain by "germs [microorganisms] of the air all that he had explained before by spontaneous generation."[2] He ignored those microorganisms within the cells of a body that can cause not only fermentation but perform other important biological functions as well.

He also taught that these minute organisms were fixed—monomorphic—entities, and he divided them into different classes, claiming that each group fermented one kind of food and another fermented another and so on. This eventually led to the theory that different bacteria caused different diseases.

This is the familiar Germ Theory of Disease, of course, and the opportunist and plagiarist was none other than the hallowed Louis Pasteur! This is an heretical idea and easy to say at this distance in time, but the facts as set forth by Ethyl Douglas Hume in her book, *Bechamp or Pasteur*, are extraordinarily well documented. Mrs. Hume spent years, apparently, poring over every scientific paper presented by (1) the chemist, Louis Pasteur, and (2) the chemist, physician, naturalist, and biologist, Professor Pierre Jacque Antoine Bechamp. As she noted their dates, it became clear that Pasteur, who, in many instances, first ridiculed Bechamp's theories, later appropriated them and took full credit for their discovery. Bechamp, on the other hand, was a brilliant scientist whose painstaking experiments and astute observations forged a theory of the nature of living bodies and their relationship to their environment that is far more salutary and, yes, holistic than Pasteur's. Heresy, again, but again, it is well documented.*

The Germ Theory

Let's look first at Pasteur's ideas and see why were so readily accepted. Aside from self-promotion, the ideas themselves were simple and easy to understand. To quote Rene Dubos of the Rockefeller Institute: "The germ theory of disease has a quality of obviousness and lucidity which makes it equally satisfying to a schoolboy and to a trained physician. A virulent microbe reaches a susceptible host, multiplies in its tissues and thereby causes symptoms, lesions and at times death. What concept could be more reasonable and easier to grasp?"[3] Or to use J. I. Rodale's summation of Pasteur's theory: "Germs live in the air, every once in a while get into a human body, multiply and cause illness. Nothing to it at all. All you have to do is kill the germs and disease is licked."[4]

Other reasons why the germ theory became popular are: (1) It fit neatly into the mechanistic theories of the universe that were popular in the 19th century. (2) It fit "human nature." Man, apparently, ever ready to avoid responsibility and place causation outside himself found an easy scapegoat in the bad little organisms that flew about and attacked him. After all, it wasn't too long ago that evil spirits had been responsible for man's ills. (3) It fit "commercial nature." When we place causation outside ourselves we create vast armies of attackers and defenders, assailants and protectors. In the case of disease causation, our protectors are such things as vaccines, drugs, and X-rays; and their administrators, medical practitioners. The possibilities for commercial exploitation are endless. Is it any wonder that the "powers that be"—conservative, well-established scientific authority—were behind Pasteur?

Nonetheless, the flaws in the fabric of the germ theory are becoming more apparent with time. Rene Dubos suggests these flaws when, after the summary statements of the theory quoted earlier, he goes on to say, "In reality, however, this view of the relation between patient and microbe is so oversimplified that it rarely fits the facts of disease. Indeed, it corresponds almost to a cult—generated by a few miracles, undisturbed by inconsistencies and not too exacting about evidence."[5]

---

*For those interested in exploring the details and more technical aspects of the experiments, observations, and arguments of these two men, I refer them to Ms Hume's book. See note 1 in the Note section of this chapter.

The Cellular Theory*

Now let us turn to Bechamp and his theories. As we proceed you will notice that Bechamp's ideas are almost the inverse of Pasteur's. In essence, Bechamp's theories are as follows:

The smallest units of living matter are what cytologists have called "cell granules," which Bechamp sometimes referred to as "granulations of the protoplasm." "Molecular granulations" and "scintillating corpuscles" are some of the names earlier researchers gave them. Bechamp called these organisms "microzymas" from the Greek meaning "small ferments" because they induce fermentation. Not all cell granules are microzymas, however. Microzymas are identifiable because they have some structure and are autonomous. They are the antecedents of cells and "the fundamental unit of the corporate organism."[6] Every living being has arisen from the microzyma and "every living being is reducible to the microzyma."[7] To get an idea of their size we might say that they are to the cell what an electron is to an atom.

Microzymas are constantly developing into bacteria. In fact, bacteria are an evolutionary form of microzymas—actually microzymas fully grown. They develop from the cells of the host organism when that organism dies. So-called virulent or pathogenic bacteria are generated by decaying matter, their function being to reduce (decompose) matter back to its constituent elements. When their job is finished they become microzymas again. Pathogenic bacteria could be thought of as nature's undertakers or clean-up crew.

The microorganisms known as "disease germs" are either "diseased" microzymas, as Bechamp called them, or their evolutionary bacterial forms. "In a diseased body a change of function in the microzymas may lead to a morbid bacterial evolution."[8] If tissue is healthy the microzymas will function to support the life and integrity of the cells; if the cells have been damaged they will produce morbid or diseased microzymas which may evolve into pathogenic (disease-producing) bacteria. In short, the microzyma has two functions: to build or to disintegrate tissue.** Another way of thinking about the function of

---

*My term.
**The physiological analog is "anabolic" which refers to constructive metabolism and "catabolic" which refers to destructive metabolism. Constructive or anabolic metabolism refers to the process of converting substances into complex compounds; catabolic metabolism refers to the process of converting tissue from a higher to a lower level of complexity or specialization. The former is constructive and proliferative; the latter releases energy from stored resources. Both processes are necessary to life; good health results from a balance of these two processes.

We might carry this further and parallel these processes with the yin and yang of Taoism. Anabolic metabolism would be yang because it consolidates energy into matter. Catabolic metabolism would be yin because it releases energy from matter.

microzymas is: they secrete ferments which aid digestion and when they encounter dead or damaged cells they evolve into bacteria.

Bechamp found microzymas everywhere—innumerable in healthy tissues, and associated with various kinds of bacteria in diseased tissues. Whether microzymas become healthy and evolve into "friendly" (aiding constructive metabolism) bacteria or diseased and evolve into pathogenic bacteria depends upon the character of the medium—cellular fluids—upon which they feed. That is, the character of the "soil"—health or unhealth of the host organism—determines the character of the microorganismic life within it. Bodies in which pathogenic bacteria form are not healthy; merely fighting and killing bacteria will not bring health, for the condition which gave rise to the bacteria will do so again.

Bechamp showed that bacteria function in whatever medium they find themselves, even changing their shapes as well as their function to accord with that medium. In comparing Pasteur's understanding of bacteria with Bechamp's, J.I. Rodale gives us this illustration: "Pasteur might have commented, while looking into a microscope 'Ah, here is the bacteria that ferments beer and this is its shape.' Bechamp might have commented, 'Here is a bacteria fermenting beer. In beer it takes on this shape.' "[9] In other words, bacteria are pleomorphic (form changing) rather than monomorphic (form fixed). They *reflect* the conditions in which they find themselves rather than create those conditions.

Modern Medicine, under the spell of the germ theory, tells us that for every disease there is a disease entity—an individual bacteria shaped in a particular way—that causes a particular disease. Bechamp showed through innumerable experiments that not only is the germ we associate with a particular disease a product and not the cause of the disease, but also that what some researchers would call different species of bacteria are really different stages of microzymian evolution into their bacterial forms. Let's look at a few of Bechamp's experiments which illustrate some of the ideas we have been discussing.

Working in a laboratory where he could get material from the nearby hospital of the Medical University of Montpellier, Bechamp and his colleagues examined a cyst that had been excised from a liver. They found microzymas in all stages of development —isolated, associated, elongated; in short, bacteria. One of Bechamp's medical pupils demonstrated that the contents of a blister included microzymas and that these evolve into bacteria. They consistently found microzymas and many forms of bacteria in various phases of development in diseased tissue.

One day an accident victim was brought to the hospital and his arm amputated. The amputation was performed between seven and eight hours after the accident and the amputated arm carried immediately to the laboratory of one of Bechamp's colleagues, Dr. Estor. When Drs. Bechamp and Estor examined the arm they found all the signs of gangrene. Under the microscope they saw microzymas associated and in chaplets (strung like beads) but no actual bacteria. Because the changes brought about by the injury had progressed so rapidly, bacteria did not have time to develop. They were merely in the process of formation. "This evidence against bacteria as the origin of the mortification was so convincing that Professor Estor at once exclaimed: 'Bacteria cannot be the cause of gangrene; they are the effects of it' "[10] We might say that while Pasture taught that germs cause disease, Bechamp taught that disease generates germs.

Years earlier, when he was developing his theories, Bechamp performed a number of experiments which proved that bacteria are indigenous to the organism and that airborne organisms need have nothing to do with their appearance in the tissues. In one experiment, he preserved the carcass of a cat in a bed of pure chalk (carbonate of lime) prepared in such a way that air would continually be renewed without permitting the intrusion of dust or microorganisms. At the end of six and a half years he removed the chalk and found nothing but fragments of bone and dry matter. There was no odor, nor was the artificial chalk discolored. Under the microscope Bechamp found microzymas swarming by the thousands in that portion of the lime where the cat's body had rested.

Repeating the experiment, Bechamp buried the carcass of a kitten; a case containing the kitten's liver; and another case containing the heart, lungs, and kidneys. This time he took even greater precaution to exclude airborne organisms. At the end of seven years he found in the bed of artificial chalk near the remains of the organs not only microzymas swarming but also well-formed bacteria. Because this second experiment had to be transported from the warmer climate of Montpellier to the colder climate of Lille a little over a year after it was begun, the destruction of the carcass was less advanced than in the previous experiment. Hence, the bacteria had not yet reverted back to microzymas as they had in the previous experiment.[11]

These two experiments confirmed the ideas suggested to Bechamp by many earlier experiments and observations. Some of the lessons learned were: (1) After the death of an organ its cells disappear, but in their place remain myriads of microzymas. (2) Microzymas can live on indefinitely after the decay of the plant or animal bodies they originally built up. Microzymas are the only nontransitory elements of the organism. (3) Microzymas are builders of plant and animal cells, which evolve into bacteria upon the death of the plant or animal. By their nutritive processes, bacteria bring about the decomposition of plant and animal bodies and, when completed, revert back to microzymas. (4) Airborne organisms, so-called atmospheric germs, are simply microzymas or their evolutionary forms (bacteria) set free by decomposition of the plant or animal body in which they lived. (5) The microzymas Bechamp had found earlier in natural chalk buried in limestone—but not in the artificial chalk produced in his laboratory—are the survivors of the constructive cellular elements of living forms of past ages. No wonder Bechamp would say, "Nothing is the prey of death; everything is the prey of life."[12]

One of Bechamp's most seminal discoveries was that there are functional but not necessarily morphological (form) differences between the microzymas of different organs of the same animal. Later he would find that there are functional differences in the microzymas of: (1) the same organs and tissues of the same animal at different ages, (2) the blood and tissues of different species, and (3) the blood and tissues of different individuals of the same species. Because microzymas of different species are functionally different, each species has diseases peculiar to it. Certain diseases are not transmissible from one species to another and often not from one individual to another even of the same species.

Implications

What implications do these ideas have for the theory and practice of vaccination? If germs are the result—one of the symptoms—of disease and not its cause, then killing, weakening, or otherwise "treating" germs will not prevent or cure disease. It is true, however, that inoculation with a specific disease germ can produce a specific disease, sometimes one associated with the specific bacteria that was injected. In one of Bechamp's experiments he inoculated plants with bacteria and studied the result of this foreign intrusion. He observed increasing swarms of bacteria in the plant interiors but he "had cause to believe that these were not direct descendants of the invaders. He became convinced," according to Ms. Hume, "that the invasion from without disturbed the inherent microzymas and that the multiplying bacteria he noted in the interior of the plants were, in his words, 'the abnormal development of constant and normal organisms.' "[13] In modern terminology, the introduction of foreign organisms disturbed the homeostasis of the plant by disrupting the normal functioning of its intracellular organisms (microzymas), thus causing them to mutate into bacteria. Another way of thinking about this would be to say that the introduction of foreign matter into the body of a plant or animal constitutes an injury, and the symptoms of that injury will accord with the nature of the injury as it interacts with the nature and condition of the organism.

If germs do not cause disease, why is it that cleanliness and aseptic surgery (essentially clean surgery) brought about such dramatic reductions in hospital fatalities resulting from such complications as puerperal (childbed) fever and wound infection? Simply, when unclean or putrefying matter—conveyed by hands, dressings, or other means—contacts fresh wounds, it introduces morbid microzymas which alter the normal function of the inherent microzymas of the body.

Pasteur talked of "invaded patients" and declared the danger of morbidity and infection to arise from atmospheric particles which he later called "microbes." In Puerperal fever, for instance, the culprit was a chain-like organism he called the germ of puerperal fever. Bechamp, on the other hand, "maintained that in free air even morbid microzymas and bacteria soon lose their morbidity, and that inherent organisms are the starting point of septic and other troubles."[14]

Perhaps the best summation of the teachings of Bechamp is given by Henry Lindlahr, M.D., in the 1918 edition of his book, *Philosophy of Natural Therapeutics*. In his discussion of Bechamp, Dr. Lindlahr says, "The physical characteristics and vital activities of cells and germs depend upon the soil in which their microzymas feed, grow and multiply. Thus microzymas, growing in the soil of procreative germ plasm, develop into normal, permanent, specialized cells of the living vegetable, animal or human organism. The same microzymas feeding on morbid materials and systemic poisons in these living bodies develop into bacteria and parasites." Dr. Lindlahr adds that he was delighted to find this scientific confirmation of the philosophy of Nature Cure which claims that "bacteria and parasites cannot cause and instigate inflammation and other disease processes unless they find their own peculiar morbid soil in which to feed, grow and multiply!"[15]

Dr. Lindlahr compares cells to atoms and microzymas to electrons: "As the electrons, according to their numbers in the atom and their modes of vibration, produce upon our sensory organs the effects of various elements of matter, so the microzymas, according to the medium or soil in which they live, develop into various cells and germs, exhibiting distinctive structure and vital activities." He suggests that the mysteries of heredity are explainable by Bechamp's theory: "If the microzymas are the spores, or seeds of cells, it is possible to conceive that these infinitesimal, minute living organisms may bear the impress of the species and of racial and family characteristics and tendencies, finally to reappear in the cells, organs and nervous system of the adult body."[16]

Florence Nightingale, the great pioneer of nursing, noted along with Drs. Creighton, Farr, and others that infectious diseases replace each other according to the varying degrees of unhealthiness of the living conditions of the people. For instance, in his *History of Epidemics in Britain*, Dr. Creighton suggests that plague was replaced by typhus and smallpox; and, later on, measles—insignificant before the middle of the 17th century—began to replace smallpox.

Regarding the germ theory, Florence Nightingale remarked, "Is it not living in a continual mistake to look upon diseases, as we do now, as separate entities, which must exist, like cats and dogs, instead of looking upon them as conditions, like a dirty and clean condition, and just as much under our own control . . . ? I was brought up to believe . . . that smallpox was a thing of which there was once a specimen in the world, which went on propagating itself in a perpetual chain of descent, just as much as that there was a first dog (or pair of dogs), and that smallpox would not begin itself anymore than a new dog would begin without there having been a parent dog. Since then I have seen with my eyes and smelt with my nose smallpox growing up in first specimens, either in close rooms or in overcrowded wards, where it could not by any possibility have been 'caught,' but must have begun. Nay, more, I have seen diseases begin, grow up and pass into one another. Now dogs do not pass into cats. I have seen, for instance, with a little overcrowding, continued fever grow up, and with a little more, typhoid fever, and with a little more, typhus, and all in the same ward or hut. For diseases, all experience shows, are adjectives, not noun substantives." She also said, "There are no specific diseases: there are specific disease conditions."[17]

MORE LOST CHAPTERS

Is there any recent research which supports Bechamp's theory that: (1) life is based on some elementary organizing energy and while this energy may take many different forms—humans, animals, insects, plants, micro-organisms—the basic material is the same and (2) disease arises from a disturbance of the normal functioning of these primal units of energy within the organism? And what about the idea that this organizing energy is contained in the "spores" or seeds of cells—to use Dr. Lindlahr's terms—which are functionally programmed for the specific organ, person, and species of which they are a part and which they helped build? What implications does this have for our practice of injecting material (microzymas) from one species into the bloodstream of another as in vaccination?

Let's begin with the idea that bacteria are not fixed—mono-morphic—entities as the germ theory insists they are, but are in fact, form changing or pleomorphic. The work of Dr. E. C. Rosenow is, as far as I know, the earliest record we have of the corroboration of Bechamp's theories. In 1910, at the Mayo Biological Laboratories, Dr. Rosenow began a series of experiments in which he took bacterial strains from many different disease sources, including puerperal sepsis, ar-thritis, tonsillitis, and cow's milk, and put them into one culture of uniform media. "After a while, there was no difference between the germs; they became all one class. Dr. Rosenow therefore concluded there was no particularly fixed species of different germs and they all had the capacity to change their structure with the changes in their nutriments."[18]

The results of his studies were published in 1914 in the *Journal of Infectious Diseases*, Volume 14, pages 1–32. Rosenow demonstrated that "simple bacterial forms like streptococci (pus germs) could be made to assume all of the characteristics of pneumococci (pneumonia germs) simply by feeding them on pneumonia virus and making other minor modifications in their environment. And when Rosenow reversed the procedure and fed pneumonia germs on pus, they quickly changed into streptococci. Many other experiments were carried on, and in every instance, the germs, regardless of type, changed into other types when their food and environment were altered."[19] In other words, Rosenow found that various strains of bacteria "or what one might call sub-sub species of them, could when suitably treated, become any of the other strains."[20]

Dr. Rosenow wrote in his 1914 article, "It would seem, therefore, that focal infections are no longer to be looked upon merely as a place of entrance of bacteria but as a place where conditions are favorable for them to acquire the properties which give them a wide range of affinities for various structures."[21] "The truth of this idea has been demonstrated in countless instances in sanitary practices," William Miller tells us. "When typhoid fever was discovered to come with con-taminated water, pure water quickly eliminated typhoid. The same is true of puerperal fever which killed so many women in childbirth. Though Semmelweiss had a hard time convincing physicians they were spreading the disease with their contaminated hands and instruments, puerperal fever was eliminated as soon as such sources of infection were removed."[22]

Cash Asher tells us that other bacteriologists have verified Rosen-

TABLE 1. TWO THEORIES OF DISEASE

GERM THEORY	CELLULAR THEORY
1. Disease arises from micro-organisms outside the body.	1. Disease arises from micro-organisms within the cells of the body.
2. Micro-organisms are generally to be guarded against.	2. These intracellular micro-organisms normally function to build tissue and assist in the metabolic processes of the body.
3. The function of micro-organisms is constant.	3. The function of these micro-organisms changes when the host organism dies or is injured, which injury may be mechanical or chemical.
4. The shapes and colors of micro-organisms are constant.	4. Micro-organisms change their shapes and colors to reflect the medium upon which they feed.
5. Every disease is associated with a particular micro-organism.	5. Every disease is associated with a particular condition.
6. Micro-organisms are primary causal agents.	6. Micro-organisms become pathogenic as the health of the host organism deteriorates. Hence, the condition of the host organism is the primary causal agent.
7. Disease can "strike" anybody.	7. Disease is built by unhealthy conditions.
8. To prevent disease we have to "build defenses."	8. To prevent disease we have to create health.

ow's findings and mentions "two New York researchers who reported transforming cocci, the round berry-shaped type of bacteria, into bacilli, the long, rod-shaped species." In the course of their experiments they discovered that "bacteria found in the primary stages of pus formation are invariably the streptococci, while in the later stages as the blood cells undergo more and more disintegration and the chemistry is altered, the 'streps' change into staphylococcus. These germs do not maintain their structural identity in an alien medium. . . . Denied their exclusive type of food, moved from their natural habitat, and fed on other kinds of food, they quickly change into forms native to their new surroundings."[23] Cash Asher likens this transformation of germs from one type to another to a mouse slowly changing into an opossum, this adaptability being characteristic of life in the microscopic world.

In the latter third of her book, particularly in Chapter 14, Ms. Hume describes later researchers who have confirmed Bechamp's theories. A few examples are the following:

> On the 8th of April, 1914, the *Daily News* of London carried this story:
> "Mme. Victor Henri, the lady bacteriologist, has made one of the most important discoveries in that branch of research for many years. She has, by subjecting bacteria to the action of ultra-violet rays, succeeded in creating a new species of bacteria from a species already known. The experiment was made with the anthrax bacillus, which from a rod-shape was transformed into a spherical coccus.[24]

A Frenchman, M. V. Galippe, carried out experiments on fruit and animal tissues which were reported in the *Bulletin de l'Academie de Médicine*, Paris, July 1917, No. 29. In experimenting with apples he found that he could induce the appearance of microorganisms from the biological activity of the microzymas by subjecting the apples to mechanical trauma such as contusions, etc. In the case of wounds—specifically war wounds—he found that not only do the crushed tissues of the wound favor the appearance and evolution of certain intracellular elements (bacteria and microzymas), but the crushed tissues and extravasated blood "may give birth directly without foreign collaboration, to infectious elements, so that an absolutely aseptic projectile is capable of infecting a wound solely by its mechanical action in starting the abnormal evolution of the living intracellular elements already present."[25]

Again we see that micro-organisms from the outside are not necessary to initiate the disease process, only injury of some sort. "In Pidoux' happy words: 'Disease is born of us and in us,' "[26] Bechamp reminds us. And like Bechamp, Galippe pointed out that microzymas are indestructible: "Neither glycerine, nor alcohol, nor time destroy the microzymas of the tissues. These different agents can only diminish or suspend their activity. They are endowed with perennial life."[27]

A reprint of speeches in the House of Lords (February 2, 1944) records a moving and interesting tribute to the work of Bechamp, given by Lord Geddes. Among other things, Lord Geddes said that he had seen and examined the little bodies under a microscope and had observed the "most extraordinary differences between people fed in different ways and in different states of health."[28]

But, perhaps the most remarkable confirmation of Bechamp's ideas comes from the research of Dr. Royal Raymond Rife of San Diego, California, who for many years built and worked with light microscopes which possessed "superior ability to attain high magnification with accompanying high resolution."[29] "With his 150,000 power microscope that made live germs visible (and) as clear as a cat in your lap,* Rife showed that . . . by altering the environment and food supply, friendly germs such as colon bacillus can be converted into pathogenic germs such as typhoid."[30] (This process is reversible.) Experiments conducted in the Rife Laboratories established the fact that "the virus of cancer, like the viruses of other diseases, can be easily changed from one form to another by means of altering the media upon which it is grown. With the first change in media, the B. X. virus becomes considerably enlarged although its purplish-red color remains unchanged. Observation of the organism with an ordinary microscope is made possible by a second alteration of the media. A third change is undergone upon asparagus base media where the B. X. virus is transformed from its filterable state into cryptomyces pleomorphia fungi, these fungi being identical morphologically both macroscopically and microscopically to that of the orchid and of the mushroom. And yet a forth change may be said to take place when this cryptomyces pleomorphia, permitted to stand as a stock culture for the period of metastasis, becomes the well-known mahogany-colored Bacillus Coli. . . . [B]y altering the media—four parts per million per volume—the pure culture of mahogany-colored Bacillus Coli becomes the turquoise-blue Bacillus Typhosus."[31] Simply stated, this means that the virus of cancer can be easily changed into

---

*In the 1920s, Rife designed and built five microscopes with a range of magnification from 5,000 to 50,000 diameters at a time when the best laboratory microscopes in use could achieve no more than 2,000 diameters of magnification. The most powerful of the Rife microscopes was the Universal Microscope with a magnification of 60,000 diameters and a resolution of 31,000 diameters as against 2,000 to 2,500 diameters in common use in that day.

The new electron microscopes have resolutions up to 20,000 or 25,000 diameters and magnifications up to 100,000 to even 200,000 diameters; however, the disadvantage of the electron microscope is that because the tiny living organisms put in it are in a vacuum and are bombarded by a virtual hailstorm of electrons they undergo protoplasmic changes and cannot be seen in their living state. The Rife microscope did not have this disadvantage; Rife was able to look at organisms in their living state. (See notes 20 and 29.)

the type of bacteria that normally inhabits the colon, and it can also be changed into the destructive bacteria of typhoid simply by slightly altering the media in which it is grown.

> It is Dr. Rife's belief that all microorganisms fall into one of not more than ten individual groups . . . and that any alteration of artificial media or slight metabolic variation in tissues will induce an organism of one group to change over into any other organism included in that same group, it being possible, incidentally to carry such changes in media to tissues to the point where the organisms fail to respond to standard laboratory methods of diagnosis. These changes can be made to take place in as short a period of time as forty-eight hours.[32]

Dr. Rife, himself, said: "In reality, it is not the bacteria themselves that produce the disease, but we believe it is the chemical constituents of these micro-organisms enacting upon the unbalanced cell metabolism of the human body that in actuality produce the disease. We also believe if the metabolism of the human body is perfectly balanced or poised, it is susceptible to no disease."[33] As a result of his studies, Rife stated: "We have in many instances produced all the symptoms of a disease chemically in experimental animals without the inoculation of any virus or bacteria into their tissues."[34] Again, "germs" are part of the disease process rather than the instigator of this process.

What about microzymas? The Universal Microscope, the most powerful Rife scope, made it possible to view the "interior of the 'pin point' cells, those cells situated between the normal tissue cells and just visible under the ordinary microscope, and to observe the smaller cells which compose the interior of these pin point cells. When one of these smaller cells is magnified, still smaller cells are seen within its structure, and when one of the still smaller cells, in its turn, is magnified, it, too, is seen to be composed of smaller cells. Each of the sixteen times this process of magnification and resolution can be repeated, it is demonstrated that there are smaller cells within the smaller cells . . . ."[35] Are these new cells within cells the microzymas of Bechamp?

"A new view of the nature of viruses is emerging. They used to be thought of solely as foreign intruders—strangers to the cells they invade and parasitize. But recent findings, including the discovery of a host-induced modification of viruses, emphasize more and more the similarity of viruses to hereditary units such as genes. Indeed, some viruses are being considered as bits of heredity in search of chromosomes," writes Dr. S. E. Luria in *Scientific American*.[36]

Dr. Lewis Thomas reaffirms this idea: "The viruses, instead of being single minded agents of disease and death, now begin to look more like mobile genes."[37] In commenting upon Dr. Luria's article, Dr. Morton Biskind says, "I would carry this thought one step further to describe viruses as aberrant nucleo-proteins which may arise in the chemically or physically damaged cell, or when introduced from without, are capable of displacing normal nucleoproteins. Just as the cell can produce its normal nucleoproteins, it now reproduces the aberrant molecules."[38] Are these nucleoproteins microzymas? Bechamp believed that damaged cells produced morbid or diseased microzymas. Dr. Biskind calls these "aberrant nucleoproteins."

Dorland's Medical Dictionary, 20th edition, defines nucleoprotein as "the conjugated protein found in the nuclei of cells. . . . It is the most important constituent of nuclei and chromatin." Could Dr. Biskind be referring to those most basic units of heredity, the DNA and RNA molecules? The DNA and RNA molecules are both forms of nucleic acids that are localized especially in the cell nuclei. Henry Lindlahr suggested that microzymas are the spores or seeds of cells, and Ethyl Douglas Hume referred to them as "Life's Primal Architects" when she wrote a pamphlet by that name.

When Professors Bechamp and Estor were working together, they observed that cell granules (microzymas) associate and develop into threadlike forms. They were no doubt observing different stages of mitosis or cell division and the development of chromatin threads. Since Bechamp earlier observed these rod-like groupings of microzymas, which now go by the name of chromosomes, my guess is that Bechamp's theories of microzymas have been incorporated into the theories of DNA and RNA as molecular units of heredity.

A hitherto unknown function of RNA has recently been discovered. Scientists have found that "RNA does more than simply carry genetic instructions and help assemble proteins for the vital processes of life." It also "serves as an enzyme, or biological catalyst, that governs some of the chemical reactions necessary for those life processes." In fact, RNA acts as a class of enzymes, those "substances that regulate the chemical activities of every living cell." The scientists, according to this article, "believe their findings eventually might help them better understand the origin of life."![39] Shades of Bechamp! My guess was apparently right.

What are viruses and are they related to genes as Drs. Luria and Thomas suggest? Could they be the microzymas Bechamp spoke of? Could they be the smaller and more numerous microzymas Bechamp observed when bacteria revert back to their original microzymian state?

Or are they the toxic by-products of bacteria as many researchers believe?[40] Since viruses are much smaller than bacteria—and can grow in the cells of animals, plants, or bacteria and are unable to grow on artificial media—I tend to think they are the ultra small microzymas Bechamp spoke of. This would seem to be true particularly when bacteria can be caused "under the right conditions of culture, to metamorphize [sic] into forms small enough to pass through filters just like viruses."[41] Since the word *virus*, however, means "poison" in Latin and is generally applied to any microscopic agent injurious to living cells, viruses could be toxic by-products of bacteria, morbid microzymas, or both.

Vaccination Revisited 1

Dr. Biskind refers to aberrant nucleoproteins. What causes them to be aberrant or atypical? As we saw earlier—and Dr. Biskind concurs—morbidity may arise from a physically or chemically damaged cell. If we think of nucleoproteins as microzymas, we remember that one way of damaging a cell is to introduce microzymas from one species into the blood of another species, or even from one organ of an animal into another organ of the same animal. In the words of Bechamp:

> "The most serious, even fatal, disorders may be provoked by the injection of living organisms into the blood; organisms which, existing in the organs proper to them, fulfill necessary and beneficial functions—chemical and physiological—but injected into the blood, into a medium not intended for them, provoke redoubtable manifestations of the gravest morbid phenomena. . . . Microzymas, morphologically identical, may differ functionally, and those proper to one species or to one center of activity cannot be introduced into an animal of another species, nor even into another center of activity in the same animal, without serious danger.[42]

If the injection of microzymas from one species to another or from one organ to another is hazardous, how much more hazardous it must be to inject foreign species of microzymas that are in a diseased or morbid condition. We are talking, of course, about some of the "foreign proteins," referred to in Chapter 2, which are the main constituents of vaccines.

We also discussed in Chapter 2 Dr. Simpson's discovery that immunizations may seed the body with RNA to form proviruses that, under proper conditions, can become activated and cause a variety of diseases including rheumatoid arthritis, multiple sclerosis, lupus erythematosus, Parkinson's disease, and cancer. He called these proviruses "molecules in search of a disease." We also pointed out that scientists have recently discovered that biological substances entering directly in the bloodstream may become part of our genetic material. As early as 1929, Dr. W. H. Manwaring, professor of bacteriology and experimental pathology at Stanford University warned against this:

> There is ground for believing that the injected germ proteins hybridize with the body proteins to form new tribes, half animal and half human, whose characteristics and effects cannot be predicted. . . . Even non-toxic bacterial substances sometimes hybridize with serum albumins to form specific poisons which continue to multiply, breed and cross-breed ad infinitum, doing untold harm as its reproductivity may continue while life lasts.[43]

A contemporary researcher might say it this way: All living organisms, including bacteria and viruses, contain genetic material (DNA or RNA). In fact, live viruses themselves are genetic messages. Live bacteria and viruses can transfer their genetic information to plant and animal cells, including human cells, which are then taken up by other cells in the body. (Plant and animal cells shed DNA.)[44] "Although the body generally will not make antibodies against its own tissues, it appears that slight modification of antigenic character of tissues may cause it to appear foreign to the immune system and thus a fair target for antibody production."[45] Thus vaccination lays the foundation for autoimmune diseases and other disorders of the immune system such as rheumatoid arthritis, rheumatic fever, lupus erythematosus, scleroderma, and periarteritis nodosa (inflammation of tissues around an artery, systemic infection, and pain around the nerves and muscles). It is reasonable to assume that our contemporary "epidemic" of allergies has at least some of its roots in the practice of vaccination.

Vaccination Revisited 2

> *Fillet of a fenny snake,*
> *In the cauldron boil and bake;*
> *Eye of newt and toe of frog,*
> *Wool of bat and tongue of dog,*
> *Adder's fork and blind-worm's sting,*
> *Lizard's leg and howlet's wing,*
> *For a charm of pow'rful trouble,*
> *Like a hell-broth boil and bubble.*
> SECOND WITCH, "MACBETH," IV: 1

Besides microorganisms that are foreign to the body, vaccines also contain other ingredients that are foreign to the body. Public health worker Carol Horowitz points out that "most parents who are trying to feed their children properly would not let them eat a food which contained any of the many ingredients of immunizations."[46] In Chapter 2 we mentioned some of these ingredients such as formaldehyde, mercury, and aluminum phosphate. Formaldehyde, which is commonly used to embalm corpses, is a known carcinogen. Mercury is a toxic heavy metal and aluminum phosphate is a toxin used in deodorants. Some of the other toxic ingredients Carol Horowitz lists are: phenol (carbolic acid), alum (a preservative), and acetone (a volatile solvent used in finger nail polish remover which can easily cross the placental barrier). Other decomposing animal proteins besides those mentioned in Chapter 2 are: (1) pig or horse blood, (2) cow pox pus, (3) rabbit brain tissue (see next chapter), (4) dog kidney tissue, and (5) duck egg protein.

A more graphic description of some of the more noxious materials in specific vaccines can be found in the literature of the British National Anti-Vaccination League: "Materials from which vaccines and serums are produced: (1) rotten horse blood, for diphteria toxin and antitoxin; (2) pulverized felt hats for tetanus serum; (3) sweepings from vacuum cleaners, for asthma and hayfever serums; (4) pus from sores on diseased cows for smallpox serums; (5) mucous from the throats of children with colds and whooping cough, for whooping cough serum; (6) decomposed fecal matter from typhoid patients for typhoid serum."[47]

Is it too impudent to suggest that man has long had a love affair with decomposing animals proteins, noxious potions that would ward off the demons of ill fortune? From the witches of old to modern medicine, man seems to be held captive by the notion that the ingestion of noxious substances protects him from the caprices of some threatening external agent. Is it too impertinent to suggest that the filth that once beset man from open sewers and unwashed clothes and bodies has returned in a new and different guise—the hypodermic needle?

NOTES

1. Ethyl Douglas Hume, *Bechamp or Pasteur? A Lost Chapter in the History of Biology*, The C. W. Daniel Company Limited, Saffron Walden; Essex, England, 1947. Subtitle of Ms. Hume's book.
2. Ibid., p. 60.

3. Rene Dubos, "Second Thoughts on the Germ Theory," *Scientific American*, May 1955, p. 31.
4. J.I. Rodale, "Bechamp or Pasteur," *Prevention* Aug. 1956, p. 69.
5. Dubos, op. cit., p. 31.
6. Hume, op. cit., p. 148.
7. Ibid., p. 112.
8. Ibid., p. 148.
9. Rodale, op. cit., p. 61.
10. Hume, op. cit., p. 118.
11. Ibid., pp. 109–11.
12. Ibid., p. 78.
13. Ibid., p. 122.
14. Ibid., p. 167.
15. Ibid., p. 161.
16. Ibid., p. 162.
17. Ibid., pp. 149–50.
18. William Miller, "Germs . . . Cause of Disease?" *Health Culture*, June 1955, p. 2.
19. Cash Asher, *Bacteria Incorporated*, Bruce Humphries, Inc., Boston, 1949, p. 14.
20. Christopher Bird, "What has become of the Rife Microscope?", *New Age*, March 1976, p. 43.
21. Ibid., p. 45.
22. Miller, op. cit., p. 2.
23. Asher, op. cit., pp. 14–15.
24. Hume, op. cit., p. 158.
25. Ibid., p. 159.
26. Ibid., p. 124.
27. Ibid., pp. 159–60.
28. Ibid., p. 164.
29. R. E. Seidel, M.D. and Elizabeth Winter, "The New Microscopes," *Journal of the Franklin Institute*, Feb. 1944, p. 117.
30. Royal Lee, D.D.S., "The Rife Microscope or 'Facts and Their Fate,' " Reprint No. 47, Lee Foundation for Nutritional Research, Milwaukee, Wis. (Cover article for the Seidel and Winter article referred to in note 29).
31. Seidel and Winter, op. cit., pp. 124–25.
32. Ibid.
33. Ibid., p. 126.
34. Bird, op. cit., p. 47.
35. Seidel and Winter, op. cit., pp. 123–24.

36. Salvador E. Luria, "The T2 Mystery," *Scientific American*, April 1955, p. 98.
37. Lewis Thomas, M.D., *The Lives of a Cell*, Bantam Books, New York, 1974, p. 3.
38. Morton Biskind, M.D., quoted by J. I. Rodale, "Bechamp or Pasteur," *Prevention*, Aug. 1956, p. 70.
39. "A function of RNA discovered," New York Times News Service, *Virginian-Pilot*, Dec. 17, 1983, p. A3.
40. *Organic Consumer Report*, Jan. 4, 1972.
41. Bird, op. cit., p. 43.
42. Hume, op. cit., p. 242.
43. Asher, op. cit., p. 19.
44. Harold Buttram, M.D., *The Dangers of Immunization*, The Humanitarian Publishing Co., Quakertown, Pa. 1979, pp. 26–30.
45. Ibid., p. 28, quotation from Peterson and Good, *Post Graduate Medicine, Special Issue, Connective Tissue Diseases*, May 1962, p. 422.
46. Carol Horowitz, "Immunizations and Informed Consent," *Mothering*, Winter 1983, p. 39.
47. Leonard Jacobs, "Menage," *East/West Journal*, Sept. 1977, p. 15.

6

∎

GERM FALLOUT: RABIES AND PASTEURIZATION

Theories imprint a whole view of the universe and make you look at everything through blinders.

WILLIAM CORLISS, *Brain/Mind Bulletin*

TWO LEGACIES

Theories come and theories go. Many of yesterday's theories and practices in medicine are now regarded as superstition, for example, bloodletting and the theory of humors. What will tomorrow's savants think of our preoccupation with vaccination and fighting germs? Indeed, yesterday's knowledge frequently becomes today's superstition and today's knowledge tomorrow's superstition. John Stuart Mill once said, "It often happens that the universal belief of one age—a belief from which no one was free, nor without an extraordinary effort of genius could, at that time, be free—becomes to a subsequent age so palpable an absurdity that the only difficulty is to imagine how such a thing can ever have appeared credible."[1]

Let's look at a few of the legacies of the germ theory, beginning with some of Pasteur's greatest "triumphs"—the supposed eradication of such diseases as rabies, anthrax (sheep and cattle disease), pebrine (silkworm disease) and, indirectly, undulant fever (brucellosis) by the pasteurization of milk. Since anthrax and pebrine are somewhat afield of our concern here, we shall not explore the chicanery involved in the promotion of the idea that Pasteur saved the livestock and silk industries. It is largely a repeat of the opportunism mentioned in Chapter 5, and anyone wishing more details on the subject may consult Ms. Hume's book. Consideration of the other two diseases, rabies and undulant fever, has important lessons for us since many people believe Pasteur saved the world from the ravages of milk-borne diseases and the bite of mad dogs. Let's begin with rabies.

RABIES

Rabies, according to one medical dictionary, is an infectious disease caused by a filterable virus which is communicated to man by the bite of an infected animal. Some of the symptoms listed are: choking; tetanic spasms, especially of respiration and deglutition (act of swallowing) which are increased by the attempts to drink water or even the sight of water; mental derangement; vomiting; and profuse secretion of sticky saliva. And the disease is usually fatal. No wonder Pasteur, with his anti-rabies vaccine, was so readily hailed as the savior of humanity from this frightening scourge!

Much has been made of the startling cure of nine-year-old Joseph Meister whom Pasteur "saved" from hydrophobia (rabies). The cure seems less than miraculous when we discover that several other persons, including the dog's owner, were bitten by that same dog on the same day and continued in good health without receiving Pasteur's inoculations. Other children were not so fortunate. Mathieu Vidau died seven months after being personally treated by Pasteur. Also, another child, Louise Pelletier, died after receiving the Pasteur treatment. Dr. Charles Bell Taylor, in the *National Review* for July 1890, gave a list of cases in which patients of Pasteur's had died while the dogs that had bitten them remained well.[2]

Apparently, then as now, organized medicine was using the police powers of the state to enforce obedience to its doctrines: A French postman, Pierre Rascol, along with another man was attacked by a dog supposed to be mad. Rascol was not actually bitten, for the dog's teeth did not penetrate his clothing. His companion, however, received severe bites. Rascol was forced by the postal authorities to undergo the Pasteur treatment, which he did from the 9th to the 14th of March. On the following 12th of April severe symptoms set in, with pain at the points of inoculation. "On the 14th of April he died of paralytic hydrophobia, the new disease brought into the world by Pasteur. What wonder that Professor Michel Peter complained: 'M. Pasteur does not cure hydrophobia: he gives it!' "[3] What happened to Rascol's companion who was severely bitten? He refused to go to the Pasteur Institute and remained in perfect health!

These stories could easily be dismissed as anecdotal except that there are a great many of them. An article in *The Archives of Neurology and Psychiatry* (January 1951) gives an account of two patients who became paralyzed after they had been treated by the Pasteur vaccine. A report in the *Journal of the American Medical Association* (January 14, 1956) relates that at a meeting of the Academy of Medicine in France, it was pointed out that the use of the Pasteur vaccination for rabies may be followed as long as 20 years later by a disorder called Korsakoff's psychosis, which is a state of delirium. Twenty years later! It was brought out at that same meeting that in a study of 460 patients treated with the Pasteur injection 20 died.[4]

The *Indiana State Medical Journal* (December 1950) reports the case of a man of 25 who received the Pasteur rabies treatment and became paralyzed from the waist down and died shortly thereafter. "The authors say that no one knows what causes these paralytic reactions. However, it has been definitely established, they say, that they are not caused by the rabies virus. In other words, vaccination, not rabies is the danger here. The authors go on to quote Sellers, another authority, who believes that 'not hydrophobia but rather rabiophobia is the most troublesome problem.' Fear of rabies, then is what we have to fear most."[5]

A story illustrating the power of suggestion to create sickness or health is told by Millicent Morden, M.D.:

A ten-year-old boy in town had been bitten by a dog, supposedly mad. Local newspapers reported he was dying of hydrophobia. Flocks of curious people were going to the house to enjoy the horrifying spectacle. The offer of a drink of water would throw the boy into a convulsion. If any object like a handkerchief or pencil were held near his head, he would growl, snapping at it savagely with his teeth and frothing at the mouth. He frequently uttered menacing growls like those of a vicious dog.

The student doctor hypnotized him and suggested that at 5 P.M. he would suddenly get well. He left asking that a swarm of visitors be kept out.

At 5 o'clock the boy announced that he was well and wanted

supper. The crowd now wanted to see the one who had wrought
the miracle in curing hydrophobia. All wanted to be treated
by him.[6]

This story, along with many others, tends to support statements
made by some doctors and kennel owners that rabies is an imaginary
disease. Dr. Morden said in the same radio address:

> On several occasions I entered the room where the victim was
> strapped down, and in addition, was being held during convulsions,
> by from one to six attendants. I unstrapped the victim, dismissed
> the attendants and assured the patient that there was no such dis-
> ease. Quick recovery followed.[7]

Many kennel owners report that in 30, 40, and even 50 years of working
with dogs, they have never seen a case of rabies, and that they and
their co-workers have been repeatedly bitten by dogs and have simply
washed the wound thoroughly with soap and water and that was the
end of it.[8]

Time magazine (November 19, 1951) gives some advice on what
to do if you are bitten by a dog. "It was proved eight years ago that
rabies virus can be removed from a wound more thoroughly by soap
and water than by nitric acid or any other cauterizing agents." Rabies
virus can be inactivated by: (1) Interferon, a protein substance produced
by the body and activated by parts of the B complex. (2) Vitamin C.
As we discussed in Chapter 4, vitamin C in sufficient quantities will
prevent the development of infectious disease. Fred Klenner found that
nerve type diseases such as polio and tetanus could be successfully
treated with the proper amount of vitamin C.[9] Rabies virus can be
inactivated in a test tube by the addition of vitamin C, and in 1967 a
veterinarian proved he could cure distemper with vitamin C.[10]

What is the rabies virus? The identifying bacteria are called "negri
bodies" which are found in the brain of the dead animal. These bodies,
however, are found in the brains of animals and people who have died
of causes having nothing to do with rabies. Frequently, they are not
found in the brains of animals which the experts were sure had rabies.
No wonder Dr. William Brady wrote as follows in the *Berkeley Gazette*
for September 1, 1954,

> I have never seen a case of rabies in man and I have never met a
> doctor who has seen a case, yet we know that the preventive in-
> oculation of Pasteur virus sometimes causes death. . . . The Pasteur
> treatment for rabies is a blind treatment and no one knows whether
> Pasteur treatment confers any protection against rabies. I'd never

willingly receive Pasteur treatment or give it to anyone under any conceivable circumstances, because I fear the material so injected has a disastrous effect in some instances. It is not always successful and occasionally paralysis follows its use."[11]

What is rabies? T. D. Dillon, kennel owner, said that most cases of supposed rabies are really running fits, teething fits, worm fits, sunstroke from heat exposure or hysteria caused by the dog finding himself in a strange environment such as a hostile, bustling, crowded city. Other kennel owners have suggested that the so-called rabid dog can be suffering from poor treatment, hunger, thirst, fear. At any rate, the Pasteur treatment is as unhealthy and risky for dogs as it is for humans. Mr. Dillon goes on to say that most dogs that he has known to be inoculated with the rabies serum have died from its aftereffects.[12]

Did, in fact, the incidence of hydrophobia decrease after the introduction of the Pasteur treatment? Dr. Charles W. Dulles, former lecturer at the University of Pennsylvania, said, "It has been shown by statistics that in countries where that method (the Pasteur treatment) is employed the number of deaths from hydrophobia has increased and not diminished."[13] Ethyl Douglas Hume points out that prior to the Pasteur treatment the average number of deaths per year from hydrophobia in France was 30. After the Pasteur treatment the number jumped to 45. She also discusses at length how the figures were manipulated to give the impression of "success."[14] Does this sound familiar?

What we said about the rabies virus is true for other viruses as well. The disease with which a particular virus is associated is sometimes present and sometimes not; people who have a particular virus may or may not have the disease associated with it. Several years ago I heard a psychiatrist, Dr. George Ritchie, describe in a public lecture the ubiquitousness of the polio virus. He told of a small town in Virginia (I've forgotten the name) in which doctors took a throat culture of everyone in town. Everyone had polio virus, yet less than ten percent of the population showed any symptoms. Of these, one-third had a slight cold, one-third had stiffness in limbs, and one-third died of bulbar polio.[15]

"All in all, a new look at the biological formulation of the germ theory seems warranted," Rene Dubos tells us. "We need to account for the peculiar fact that pathogenic agents sometimes can persist in the tissues without causing disease and at other times can cause disease even in the presence of specific antibodies. We need also to explain why microbes supposed to be nonpathogenic often start proliferating in an unrestrained manner if the body's normal physiology is upset. . . .

"During the first phase of the germ theory the property of virulence

TABLE 2. THE GERM THEORY *vs.* EXPERIMENTAL DATA

THE GERM THEORY*	CONTRAINDICATIONS FROM EXPERIMENTAL DATA
To be the causative agent a particular disease germ:	
1. Must be found in every case of the disease.	1. May not be found in every case of the disease.
2. Must never be found apart from the disease.	2. May frequently be found apart from the disease.
3. Must be capable of culture outside the body.	3. May be capable of culture outside the body. However, the original disease germ must be obtained from diseased tissue.
4. Must be capable of producing by injection the same disease as that undergone by the body from which the disease germs were taken.	4. May or may not produce the same disease as the body from which the disease germs were taken. For instance, the pneumococcus of pneumonia introduced into the lung of a rabbit results not in pneumonia, but septicemia.**

*The germ theory is based upon these formulations by a 19th-century German doctor, William Frederick Koch.
**Hume, *Bechamp or Pasteur?*, p. 208.

was regarded as lying solely within the microbes themselves. Now virulence is coming to be thought of as ecological. Whether man lives in equilibrium with microbes or becomes their victim depends upon the circumstances under which he encounters them. This ecological concept is not merely an intellectual game; it is essential to a proper formulation of the problem of microbial diseases and even to their control."[16]

The narrow focus on ridding ourselves and our world of harmful bacteria without considering the ecological relationships within the milieu in which they function has been disastrous in many instances. For example, antibiotics can unbalance the ecology of the body to the point where protective or beneficial bacteria are destroyed and fungus infestations, such as the recent "epidemic" of candida albicans, can result. Inflammations and increased susceptibility to infections are also possible side effects. Other serious problems can occur as well. For instance, streptomycin destroys the innervation to the balancing mechanism of the inner ear. Sulfa drugs—effective because they mobilize vitamin C from the tissues into the blood—can damage the kidneys.[17] Sulfa drugs can also cause anemia, allergies, and inflammation of the heart.[18]

Now let's take a look at milk and see what effects the narrow focus of just destroying "harmful" bacteria has had on the nutritional value and even the safety of milk.

MILK PASTEURIZATION

Pasteurization, named for Louis Pasteur, is the process of heating milk or other substances to 130 to 158 degrees Fahrenheit for 20 or 30 minutes. The new "flash" methods of pasteurizing heat the milk to 150 to 170 degrees for 15 to 22 seconds. This is done to kill pathogenic bacteria and delay the development of other bacteria. However, according to Norman Walker, D.Sc., temperatures from 190 degrees to 230 degrees Fahrenheit are required to kill pathogenic organisms such as typhoid, bacilli coli, tuberculosis, and undulant fever.[19] This, of course, would damage the milk to such an extent that no cream would rise—a drawback from a commercial standpoint.

The heat of pasteurization is enough, however, to kill the beneficial lactic acid, or souring bacteria—lactobacillus acidophilus—which help to synthesize B vitamins in the colon and hold the putrefactive bacteria in check. Raw milk will eventually curdle and clabber if allowed to sit at room temperature because the lactic acid bacteria hold the putrefactive bacteria in check. Pasteurized milk, having no such protection, will rot. Hence, the irony of pasteurization is that it destroys the germicidal properties of milk. While pasteurization cuts down the bacterial count temporarily, the count soon exceeds the figure prior to pasteurization, because bacteria multiply more rapidly in pasteurized milk than in raw milk. Royal Lee, D.D.S., claims many cases of undulant fever can be found in communities where all milk is pasteurized.[20] Salmonella food poisoning which affected over 500 people in Illinois and Iowa during March and April, 1985, was traced to pasteurized milk.[21]

What causes undulant fever? It has been shown to be a deficiency disease curable in both man and animal by the administration of trace minerals.[22] Particularly important are manganese and magnesium.[23]

The primary commercial advantages of pasteurizing milk are: (1) It enables the farmer to be dirty. Standards for certified dairy herds and milk handlers are considerably higher than those for herds whose milk is to be pasteurized; hence, it costs more to make clean, raw dairy products. (2) It is a convenience for the grocer as well as the farmer. Although raw milk will generally keep longer than pasteurized milk, if it is not produced under sanitary conditions it will begin to curdle sooner than pasteurized milk will begin to smell rotten. Hence, pasteurization can hide staleness and give milk a longer shelf life.

How does the heat of pasteurization affect the nutritional value of milk? Heating any food above 122 degrees Fahrenheit destroys enzymes, those biochemical transformers that trigger the thousands of chemical processes going on in our bodies all the time. One of the functions of enzymes is to release nutrients in the food we eat. The heat of pasteurization destroys the enzyme phosphatase, which is necessary for the assimilation of calcium. Some researchers claim that as much as 50 percent of the calcium in pasteurized milk is not utilized by the body.*[24]

Other food factors and skeletal structures adversely affected by pasteurization as well as diseases promoted by this practice are:

(1) *Vitamins:* The loss of fat-soluble vitamins such as A and E may run as high as two-thirds. The loss of water soluble vitamins such as B and C can run from 38 percent to 80 percent. The vitamin C loss usually exceeds 50 percent.[25]

(2) *Minerals:* Twenty percent of available iodine is lost by volatilization. There is loss of availability of other minerals in varying degrees.[26]

(3) *Thirty-eight or more food factors* are changed or destroyed, including protein and hormones as well as the vitamins and minerals discussed. Fats are also altered by heat as well as the whole protein complex which is rendered less available for tissue repair and rebuilding.[27]

(4) *Anti-stiffness and anti-anemia factor:* Pasteurization destroys the guinea pig "anti-stiffness" (Wulzen factor) and "anti-anemia" factor in milk.[28]

(5) *X Factor:* The X factor in tissue repair is destroyed.[29]

(6) *Teeth and bones.* Children's teeth are less likely to decay on a diet supplemented with raw milk than with pasteurized milk.[30] Dr. F. M. Pottenger, Jr., who has studied the effects of raw milk on both experimental animals and people, reported that raw milk produced better bones and teeth than pasteurized milk, and that it protected against or prevented dental problems, deafness, arthritis (due to presence of the Wulzen factor), rheumatic fever, and asthma.[31]

(7) *Coronary thrombosis and arteriosclerosis.* "Dairy products fed

---

*A number of studies have pointed to widespread symptoms of calcium deficiency among Americans, and yet we are one of the highest consumers of milk and milk products in the world. (Out of 148 countries, we rank 11th in per capita milk protein consumption, according to *The New Book of World Rankings,* 1984 edition.) Could pasteurization of milk and milk products have something to do with this?

[eaten] in large amounts, including raw cream and raw butter do not produce atheroma, do not raise the blood cholesterol, while the highest grade pasteurized produce does."[32] "Pasteurization, or the heating of milk which changes the structure of protein, is a major cause of coronary thrombosis," declared Dr. J. C. Annand from Dundee, Scotland. "The consumption of heated milk protein . . . not milk fat . . . has been found to correlate historically to the high incidence of thrombosis," he added.[33]

(8) *Skeletal deformities and degenerative diseases.* Experimental animals deteriorate rapidly on pasteurized milk.

For instance, calves fed pasteurized milk die within 60 days as shown by numerous experiments.[34] Perhaps the most famous and, by now, classical experiment is the one of Dr. Francis M. Pottenger's, which was reported at the Second Annual Seminar for the Study and Practice of Dental Medicine, in Palm Springs, California, in October 1945. The report outlined the results of ten years of careful study of approximately 900 cats which were bred and studied for four and five generations. The cats were divided into six groups. The first group was fed raw meat, raw milk, and cod liver oil. The second group was fed the same except the meat was cooked. The other groups were fed raw meat and various kinds of cooked milk, i.e., pasteurized milk, evaporated milk, and sweetened condensed milk. Only the cats in the first group remained healthy throughout the experiment. The cats in the other groups suffered skeletal deformities, parasitic infestations, allergies, arthritis, reproductive failure, skin lesions, cardiac lesions, and many other degenerative conditions familiar in the literature of human medicine.

One of the more interesting features of the experiment was observing what happened in each of the pens that housed the cats after the experiment was over. The pens lay fallow for several months. Weeds sprang up in each pen, but only the pen that housed the raw meat-, raw milk-fed cats supported luxuriant growth. This led the experimenters to perform a further experiment. They planted beans in each pen and again, only the pen of the raw meat-, raw milk-fed cats supported the growth of bean plants to any real degree. Vegetation in the other pens was sparse and scraggly, being the most sparse in the pen of the sweetened, condensed milk-fed cats. These cats were the ones which showed the most marked deficiencies and degenerative changes during the experiment. (I couldn't help thinking as I read this, "This is the kind of milk, essentially, that many people feed their babies!")

The experimenters concluded: "The principles of growth and development are easily altered by heat and oxidation, which kill living cells at every stage of the life process, from the soil through the animal. Change is not only shown in the immediate generation, but as a germ plasm injury which manifests itself in subsequent generations of plants and animals."[35]

Fresh, raw milk has been successfully used as a therapeutic agent since Hippocrates who prescribed it for tuberculosis, William Campbell Douglass, M.D., reminds us. In his informative and humorous book, *The Milk of Human Kindness is not Pasteurized,* he describes many other ailments that have been successfully treated with fresh, whole, clean, raw milk. Some of these are: (1) edema, (2) obesity, (3) allergies, (4) high blood pressure, (5) psoriasis, (6) diabetes, (7) diseases of the prostate gland, (8) urinary tract infections, (9) heart and kidney disease, (10) hardening of the arteries, (11) neuresthenia, (12) arthritis, (13) gastric and duodenal ulcers, and (14) muscle cramps during pregnancy. Pasteurized milk will not work. It must be raw.[36]

FROM FRAGMENTATION TO HOLISM

The primary legacy of the germ theory is its fragmentation and narrow focus—its focus on microorganisms rather than milieu, on symptoms rather than causes, on parts rather than wholes. Our discussion of milk pasteurization is particularly illustrative of the counterproductivity of focusing on destroying the "bad guys," or life forms that appear inimical to health, while ignoring the ecological web that sustains both the "good guys" and the "bad." In the field of agriculture the same kind of tunnel vision is responsible for ever more potent pesticides that destroy not only the "bad" bugs but their natural predators as well, to say nothing of the toxic residues of the pesticides that enter the food chain and eventually the human digestive tract.

The germ theory is at least partly responsible for our obsession with pathology and our sense of alienation from the natural world, an alienation so profound we feel justified in inflicting pain and suffering upon animals to measure the course of some pathology or to obtain a new medicine or vaccine. For instance, this is how rabies vaccine was made. I say "was" because now, I hear, there is a new vaccine, but this is how it was made until at least 1947.

1. A rabbit, dog, or goat is strapped and its head held.
2. With no anesthetic, a cut is made through the skull on top of the head.
3. Skin is separated from the skull.

4. A circular saw then removes some bone.
5. A piece of the brain of a so-called rabid dog is then inserted and the skin sewed up; the animal is then placed in a cage to die a slow and horrible death.
6. In 13 to 27 days death occurs from inflammation of the brain. At death, the brain and spinal cord are removed, dried, and later mashed up in a distilled water and salt solution to which carbolic acid or chloroform is added.
7. After straining, it is ready for animal or human use.[37]

Could man's proverbial inhumanity to man have at least some of its genesis in the license he takes with his fellow creatures?

Perhaps an even more insidious legacy of the germ theory is the mind-set that sees disease as an implacable and treacherous foe, a "thief in the night" that strikes without warning and without discrimination. The universe is reduced to a battlefield and man to a warrior who must build defenses and destroy enemies. This adversarial reductionism not only erodes man's sense of harmony and relatedness to the natural world, but it is belittling to the human spirit. Sri Aurobindo, the great Hindu sage, poet, and philosopher, states the case succinctly: "I would rather die and have done with it than spend life in defending myself against a phantasmal siege of microbes. If that is to be barbarous, unenlightened, I embrace gladly my Cimmerian darkness."[38]

What would medicine be like if Bechamp's ideas had been accepted instead of Pasteur's? First, it would be health rather than disease oriented. Rather than focusing on disease symptoms, it would focus on the patient—his life-style, his temperament, his body type; his habits of eating, exercising, thinking, and feeling. Instead of classifying microorganisms and disease entities, it would classify environments and life styles; instead of fighting germs, it would focus on building healthy bodies; and in agriculture it would focus not on killing pests but on building a balanced, healthy soil which in turn produces healthy plants that don't "attract pests." (More about this later.)

Does any of this sound familiar? Yes, we are talking about holistic health, natural healing, and organic gardening—ideas whose time has come.

NOTES

1. Quoted by Clinton Miller, Hearings before the Committee on Interstate and Foreign Commerce, House of Representatives, Eighty-

Seventh Congress, Second Session on H.R. 10541, May 1962, p. 86.

2. Ethyl Douglas Hume, *Bechamp or Pasteur? A Lost Chapter in the History of Biology*, The C. W. Daniel Company Limited, Saffron Walden, Essex, England, 1947, pp. 196–98.

3. Ibid., p. 198.

4. J. I. Rodale, "Rabies, Fact or Fancy," *Prevention*, Aug. 1956, p. 52.

5. Ibid., pp. 52–53.

6. Millicent Morden, M.D., radio address, WWRL, Jan. 1947. (From a leaflet distributed by Health Research, Mokelumne Hill, Calif.)

7. Ibid.

8. *The Fraud of Rabies*, collection of statements by medical doctors, veterinarians and kennel owners distributed by the California Animal Defense and Anti-Vivisection League, Inc. (booklet undated).

9. *Southern Medicine and Surgery*, Aug. 1952, "The Vitamin and Massage Treatment for Acute Poliomyelitis," pp. 194–97. Quoted by Marilyn Garvan, "Mandatory Rabies Shots Protested," *National Health Federation Bulletin*, 1974, p. 22.

10. Ibid.

11. Rodale, pp. 50–51.

12. *The Fraud of Rabies*, op. cit.

13. Ibid.

14. Hume, op. cit. p. 200.

15. George Ritchie, M.D. "The Ego and the Holy Spirit," lecture at A.R.E., Virginia Beach, Dec. 30, 1978.

16. Rene Dubos, "Second Thoughts on the Germ Theory," *Scientific American*, May 1955, pp. 34–35.

17. Royal Lee, D.D.S., "It can Happen Here," *Nature's Path*, April 1951.

18. James and Peta Fuller, "The Other Side of the Wonder Drugs," *The American Mercury*, Lee Foundation Reprint #46 (undated).

19. Norman Walker, *Diet and Salad Suggestions*, Norwalk Laboratory, Publishing Department, St. George, Utah, 1947, p. 32.

20. Royal Lee, D.D.S., "The Battlefront for Better Nutrition," *The Interpreter*, July 15, 1950.

21. "Food Poisoning Cases in Illinois," item in "Health Notes," *Health Freedom News*, May 1985, p. 31.

22. Ed. Rupp, "What About Trace Minerals?", *Missouri Ruralist*, April 9, 1949. Also, "Are We Starving at Full Tables?" *Steel Horizons*, Vol. 12, No. 3.

23. Adelle Davis, *Let's Get Well*, Harcourt, Brace & World, Inc., New York, 1965, p. 149.

24. Elizabeth J. Broadston, "Hear Ye—Mothers!", *Let's Live*, Feb. 1955, p. 12. Also, Royal Lee, D.D.S., "Raw Food Vitamins." Address delivered before the Massachusetts Osteopathic Society Convention, Boston, May 22, 1949.

25. Linda Clark, *Stay Young Longer*, Pyramid Books, New York, 1971, p. 194. Also, "Abstracts on the Effect of Pasteurization on the Nutritional Value of Milk," Lee Foundation for Nutritional Research, Reprint #7.

26. Jean Bullit Darlington, "Why Milk Pasteurization?", *The Rural New-Yorker*, May 3, 1947, p. 4. Also Broadston, op. cit. p. 12.

27. Broadston, op. cit. p. 12.

28. Darlington, op. cit. p. 5.

29. Ibid.

30. *Lancet*, May 8, 1937, p. 1142. (Taken from Lee Foundation for Nutritional Research, Reprint #7.)

31. Clark, op. cit. pp. 194–95.

32. Francis M. Pottenger Jr., M.D., "A Fresh Look at Milk." This article first appeared in Mr. Kenan's report in the "History of Randleigh Farm." (This reprint is undated, but an article by J. F. Wischhusen and N. O. Gunderson, M.D., "The Nutritional Approach to the Prevention of Disease," in *The Science Counselor*, September 1950, refers to the book, *The History of Randleigh Farm*, 4th ed., William R. Kenan, Jr., Lockport, N.Y., 1942.)

33. *Organic Consumer Report*, Oct. 7, 1975.

34. Henry G. Bieler, M.D., *Food is Your Best Medicine*, Random House, New York, May 1969. p. 213.

35. Francis M. Pottenger, Jr., M.D., "The Effect of Heat-Processed Foods and Metabolized Vitamin D Milk on the Dentofacial Structures of Experimental Animals," *American Journal of Orthodontics and Oral Surgery*, Aug. 1946, pp. 467–85.

36. William Campbell Douglass, M.D., *The Milk of Human Kindness is not Pasteurized*, Last Laugh Publishers, Marietta, Ga. 30067, 1985, Chapter 11.

37. Millicent Morden, M.D., "Rabies Vaccine," California Animal Defense and Anti-Vivisection League, Inc., Los Angeles, Calif. (This flier is not dated but a radio address given by this same doctor and distributed by Health Research is dated Jan. 25, 1947.)

38. Sri Aurobindo, "Natural Health—or 'Science'?", *Advent*, Aug. 1953, p. 154. (Reprinted in *Health Movement Review*, March 1955.)

7

■

HOLISM, EPIDEMICS, AND PREVENTIVE "MEDICINE"

We are completely, firmly, absolutely connected with all of existence, and . . . the next evolutionary step will involve, at the least, our realizing that connection.

GEORGE LEONARD, *The Silent Pulse*

HOLISM

Is the universe a machine, a battlefield, a thought, or an organism? The metaphor we choose will organize and direct our thinking about ourselves and our relationship to the world around us. The metaphor of the universe as a thought or an organism is, of course, most compatible with the newer holistic models of reality. "Many levelled mind" (Fritjof Capra) and "a great thought" (Sir James Jeans) are some of the terms physicists have used to describe the universe. Physician Lewis Thomas sees our world as a cell. Chemist and inventor James Lovelock sees our planet as a living being whose biosphere and atmosphere are a single living system. (He terms this the "Gaia Hypothesis.")

The universe is not only alive and intelligent, but it is a web of interconnections: "Quantum interconnectedness" (John Bell) and "unbroken wholeness" (David Bohm) are again some of the terms physicists have used to describe it. In the world of microorganisms "every creature is, in some sense, connected to and dependent upon the rest," Lewis Thomas points out.[1] Nothing can be understood in isolation; everything is a part of an interrelated, interacting system according to General Systems Theory, and I would add ecology and holistic healing.

I include ecology with holistic healing because, in a sense, holistic healing is the ecological approach to understanding and working with the body. It means seeing any part only in relation to a larger whole, e.g., an organ or a function in relation to other organs and functions of the body, and the body in relation to an environment and a life style. Holism is essentially contextualism.

The contextual nature of holistic healing has come to mean studying and working with the patient as a whole—his spirit, mind, and emotions as well as his body. I avoid using the term "treating" and use instead the term "working with" because this latter implies conscious partici-pation on the part of the patient whereas the former implies passive receptivity. It is this conscious participation in the healing process that is one of the distinguishing features of holistic healing.

The mind is a central factor in any healing process. There is abun-dant evidence that belief in a therapeutic modality is a primary com-ponent of the effectiveness of that modality. Medical and anthropological literature is replete with stories of people who have been healed—and killed—by the pronouncements of witch doctors in whom they believed. "Now we know that the brain and immune system are 'hard wired' together. Not only are there direct central nervous system links which modulate the expression of immunocompetence, but immune reactions alter brain activity as well."[2] The new science of psychoneuroimmunology—the study of how the central nervous system affects the immune system—shows that the state of one's mind is re-flected by the state of one's immune system.[3] It's no longer news that stress impairs the functioning of the immune system and that emotional distress is implicated as one of the causes of disease, infectious as well as degenerative.

Can a physician regard himself as holistic who insists upon giving a patient a treatment he doesn't want? The question seems absurd on the face of it, yet there are doctors who call themselves holistic who think it not inconsistent to disregard a patient's wishes with respect to a treatment. For example, I talked with a woman from Wisconsin who told me she phoned a well-known medical doctor in the Virginia Beach area who was listed in several health care publications as a holistic doctor. He had a position of leadership in two holistic health organizations. She and her family were living in Wisconsin and were considering moving to Virginia when she phoned the doctor. She asked him if they chose him for their family doctor would he exempt the children from the state vaccination requirement? She made it clear that she had studied the matter and did not want her children vaccinated. He told her he would insist that they have at least the polio and tetanus shots!

Why are holism and coercion contradictory? Because coercion removes the patient's mind and spirit from the health or healing process. Coercion is the ultimate assertion of the ego—of hubris and separation—because it treats the other as an object. The one who coerces says in effect, "It is OK for me to manipulate you for an end that my superior knowledge, position, or power deems right."

According to Marcus Bach, the word "holism" comes from the Greek word "hololes" meaning holy, sacred, complete, and implies regarding the other as a holy being, a spiritual entity.*[4]

Holism is not new. It is actually a rebirth and a reintegration of the paradigm of holism that reigned prior to the Middle Ages. The functions of priest, teacher, and physician were considered as one, and a healer functioned in all three capacities because he worked with the whole person—the spirit (priest), the mind (teacher), the body (physician). These functions became separated during the Middle Ages with the advent of specialization, and the totality of the individual was lost.[5] Now these functions are beginning to converge, and we see the holistic healer becoming a caring teacher-partner who regards his patients as holy beings. This perception of the other as a holy being who is spiritually inseparable from ourselves is the bedrock upon which we experience reverence for all life.

If the universe is indeed more like an organism—or a thought—than a collage of disparate objects, then what is implied when a sizeable number of people manifest a similar set of symptoms within a specific space-time frame? Let's take a second look at that frightening and puzzling phenomenon known as epidemics.

EPIDEMICS AND PREVENTIVE "MEDICINE"

"When I use a word, it means just what I choose it to mean—neither more nor less," Humpty Dumpty told Alice,

LEWIS CARROLL, *Alice in Wonderland*

---

*Sometimes the word "holism" is spelled "wholism." The focus here is on the idea of wholeness, the whole person, rather than his consciousness per se or the idea that he is a holy being.

What is an epidemic? If we lived in the 14th century (around 1350) and we heard of an epidemic of plague, we would know that as many as 75 percent of the people in a given community could be affected. If we lived in the United States in the middle of the 20th century and we heard of an epidemic of polio, it could mean that as few as .02 percent (1 out of every 5,000) could be affected. Here, we will define an epidemic as a set of similar symptoms affecting a noticeable proportion of the population in a given community or communities.

Let's look at some reports of the more dramatic epidemics, both historical and current, remembering the inevitable distortions that inhere within the act of reporting. From these reports some instructive inferences can be drawn.

That Bug Going Around

The influenza epidemic of 1918 is one of the more puzzling epidemics of history. According to an article in the *Los Angeles Times*, it spread to every country of the world, killing an estimated 21 million people and sparing only the Island of St. Helena and Mauritius Island in the Indian Ocean. "Coast Guard searching parties discovered Eskimo villages in remote, inaccessible Alaskan regions that were wiped out to the last adult and child. A British army officer who traveled through northern Persia in 1919 brought a report that in village after village there were no survivors."[6]

"New York City counted 851 deaths in a single day. Chicago did not have enough hearses, and bodies stacked up in the morgues." Dr. Ralph Chester Williams, a former assistant U.S. surgeon general, recalls those fearful days of the 1918 influenza epidemic: "We were swamped with soldiers, sailors, marines and coast guardsmen. They would just collapse in streets downtown and were brought out to us. . . . There was a Marine sergeant. He was brought in unconscious and in three hours that man was dead. Just like that. It was common knowledge that between 400 and 500 people were dying in Chicago each day. More people were dying than could be buried."[7]

The cause, or causes, of this tragedy has been speculated upon but never, to my knowledge, fully resolved. A discussion of this epidemic in the *Journal of the American Medical Association* (Sept. 11, 1920, page 755) points out that "those under 35 died in appalling numbers; those over 55 seemed to be relatively safe." This is a reversal of the age incidence of previous influenza epidemics in which the age group most affected was over 55.

What would cause this age incidence reversal? What was common to people under 35 that was not common to people over 55? Vaccination comes immediately to mind, especially vaccination against typhoid which was introduced in 1909. People under 35, servicemen as well as young women working in munitions factories, died in large numbers from influenza. They would be more inclined to be vaccinated than older segments of the population. However, throughout history plagues have nearly always followed in the wake of war, varying in intensity to the degree that the sanitary and hygienic conditions of the population were healthful or unhealthful.* The far-reaching ravages of the influenza epidemic may possibly be explained by the distribution of military campaigns in widely diversified areas. (The number of deaths attributed to this epidemic varies considerably according to reportage.)[8] Water pollution and bacterial modification of typhoid to influenza are possible causes suggested by some researchers.[9]

Whatever the cause, a relatively simple treatment proved to be remarkably effective in curing it. The treatment involved no drugs or medication of any kind and, although simple, it was time-consuming. Probably for these reasons it was not used by medical doctors.

Dr. R. Lincoln Graham, a naturopathic physician of that period and a recognized authority on hydrotherapy, discusses in his book on that subject how he treated over 400 cases of the flu without a single loss of life. He also tells how during the great diphtheria epidemic in Berlin in 1900 he treated 28 cases of diphtheria without a single fatality. He treated these cases in a clinic operated by a Dr. Guenther who, seeing the remarkable results of this treatment, tried to get the Charities Hospital to adopt it. Dr. Guenther was unsuccessful, and thousands throughout the city died.

Dr. Graham's treatment for flu consists of four basic steps: (1) No food until the disease is over. (2) A glass of water every hour, preferably spring water. (3) An enema or high-colonic irrigation every day. (4) A cold, wet pack around the chest in case of symptoms of pneumonia.

"When I first read this remarkable book," Dr. Wright, another naturopathic physician, said in reference to Dr. Graham's book, "I could scarcely believe the astounding results reported, but since I have been putting his methods into practice the results have never once been disappointing; they are almost routine." He then tells of the first time he tried Dr. Graham's method:

*"It is said that when plagues decimated millions in Europe throughout the Middle Ages, many survived by eating garlic cloves daily. They would disinfect areas by scattering the potent cloves over waste pileups." More recently, Russian doctors cured so many infections with garlic, that it has been called "Russian Penicillin." In the 1965 flu epidemic in Russia, a 500-ton emergency shipment of garlic was distributed throughout the danger areas. The government-controlled newspapers urged people to eat more garlic. (Carlson Wade, "Country Kitchen," *Better Nutrition*, March 1982, p. 30.)

"I was called to the home where a six-year-old child lay dying of pneumonia. The attending physician told me, 'This child will die before morning.' However, I began the hydrotherapy treatment and within the hour the most remarkable change took place. She had been extremely constipated, was too weak to cough up the mucous that was half choking her, and constantly moaned in pain.

"Soon the moans stopped; her bowels moved three times normally and the strangling mucous poured our of her. Her temperature gradually dropped from 104.5° to 97°, and the next morning this child was well—completely well! It taught me a great lesson and reinforced my belief in Dr. Graham's methods, which I have continued to use."[10]

How does this treatment relate to the ideas of holistic healing discussed earlier? Holism, or contextualism, can be applied to micro- as well as macroorganismic life. Lewis Thomas tells us that microbes "live together in dense, interdependent communities, feeding and supporting the environment for each other. . . . and that "We can no more isolate one from the rest, and rear it alone, than we can keep a single bee from drying up like a desquamated cell when removed from the hive."[11] Not only are bacteria "groupies," so to speak, they are also, in a sense, chameleons, reflecting an environment from which they are inseparable. Each type of bacteria "has been studied as a pure culture only by isolating it upon a specific nutrient called media," Christopher Bird tells us. "While outside a host or body, bacteria are hard to raise, or culture."[12] It is pertinent to note that to culture bacteria, dead, or decaying food must be used.[13]

What does this tell us about rhetoric that refers to "that bug going around" and germs that "attack" people? Isn't it more holistic to think of a substance—which includes microorganisms—that enters the ecological system of either a single body or a community of bodies? If the substance is in a state of decay, the microorganisms will be pathogenic. To the degree that the life support system of either an individual or a community is unbalanced and toxic, to that degree will the intrusion of foreign substances accelerate pathological change. To the degree that the ecology of the body or community is balanced and free of accumulated waste material, to that degree will pathogenic bacterial processes be reversed or nullified. The hydrotherapy treatments of Drs. Graham and Wright illustrate that when the body is internally cleansed, pathogenic bacteria have nothing more to feed upon and the disease process reverses itself.

The relationship between imbalance and toxicity is perhaps best illustrated by nutrition. The current emphasis on whole, natural, unadulterated food is part of the contextual thinking that characterizes holism. When food is fragmented, it is no longer balanced and can produce toxic metabolic residues in the body. For instance, refined white sugar and flour produce toxic metabolites such as pyruvic acid and abnormal sugars containing five carbon atoms which interfere with cell respiration and eventually the functioning of a part of the body. This begins the degenerative disease process.[14]

Since any kind of adulteration produces imbalances in our bodies, we can think of purification and rebalancing as correctives that will reverse life-threatening disease processes. To rebalance is, in a sense, to purify and vice versa. In the next two sections we will see how it is possible to create imbalances in the ecosystem by introducing poisons into the system and how it is possible to compensate, to a certain extent, for the adulteration of one part of the life support system by rebalancing another part of that system.

What's Going Around?

Let's look at symptoms for a moment. Can you guess what disease entities are characterized by these symptoms?

(1) Begins with high fever and aching bones. Many cases, after about four days, develop pneumonia. The lungs of victims fill with fluid, causing death.[15]

(2) Headache, nausea, vomiting, general malaise and dizziness.[16]

(3) Sharp, recurrent pains in the muscles of the neck, thorax, and shoulders; severe headache; and disturbance in coordination with some motor and sensory disturbances.[17]

(4) Unexplained headaches, great thirst, nausea, vomiting, abdominal cramps, diarrhea, seizures that are not epileptic.[18]

The first group of symptoms were the symptoms of the 1918 flu epidemic. The second and third group of symptoms are the symptoms of pesticide poisoning: the second being the early symptoms of dieldrin poisoning, and the third being typical of mysterious "diseases" that occur in heavily sprayed areas, according to chemist and agricultural expert, Leonard Wickenden. The fourth group of symptoms are some of the symptoms of early fluoride poisoning which can occur even at the recommended concentration of one part per million for municipal drinking water.

"In a recent Hearing, before a Pesticide Committee, a noted medical doctor (Granville Knight), stated under oath that Monitor-4 is of the same chemical family as the defoliants used in Vietnam; the waves of so-called "Virus-X" and similar diseases . . . are caused by exposure to such agricultural chemicals; that it is impossible for doctors to diagnose the difference between London Flu, Virus Conditions, and Pesticide Poisonings!"[19]

A July 15, 1985, *U.S. News and World Report* article, "Is the Food You Eat Dangerous to Your Health?", reported that American farmers use one billion pounds of insecticides every year—nearly 4.5 pounds for every man, woman, and child in the United States. The same month I heard on the news (July 6, 1985) that 300 people had been stricken with flu-like symptoms from pesticide poisoned watermelons grown in California.

Interpreting symptoms of pesticide poisoning as "that bug going around" has been going on for well over 30 years. Dr. F. L. Mickle wrote in the *Connecticut Health Bulletin* of Jan. 1952:

> Virus diseases which appear to be increasing are coming to the foreground. They are of much greater importance in the State than formerly. For instance, almost every person you meet on the street or in the homes of your friends speaks at one time or another of having had the "virus that's going around" . . . these viruses cause distressing and incapacitating *upper respiratory symptoms* often accompanied by *diarrhea* and *vomiting*.[20] (italics mine)

The above are some of the symptoms of DDT and related pesticide poisoning. So-called "infectious" hepatitis has been linked to chlordane poisoning,[21] and, as I pointed out earlier in Chapter 4, epidemics of poliomyelitis have been linked to DDT poisoning. Although I am tempted to say that viruses appear sometimes to be the all-purpose dodge, "it should be pointed out that not only may a toxic agent which damages a particular organ simulate infectious disease, but the damaged organ is more susceptible to transmissible agents, if exposure occurs."[22]

How can injury be repaired? What therapy supports the health and vitality of the whole person? What remedial measures can be taken to support the health of the soil and the environment after they have been damaged by toxic agricultural chemicals? The first step, of course, is to eliminate further exposure to the toxin. In the case of injured people, a number of doctors have found the "administration of intensive, complete and persistent nutritional therapy is essential" to repair liver damage. This includes vitamins, liver supplements, lipotropic (fat utilizing) factors, and a high protein diet.[23] To heal the soil, organic composting and mulching can be applied.

Are there any preventive measures we can take *before* exposure to toxic substances? "Medical literature is filled with reports on studies which show that vitamin C can neutralize and destroy toxins in the body and increase the body's resistance to virtually any bacterial toxins as well as drug insults," Dr. Paavo Airola informs us.[24] As with other poisons, immunizations destroy vitamin C in the body. Along with high doses of vitamin C, Dr. Airola recommends garlic, vitamins A and the B complex, the minerals zinc and calcium, as well as certain herbs for several weeks *prior to* and *after* immunizations of infants or children. He recommends this to parents who, after examining the evidence, *choose* to have their children immunized.[25]

In his fascinating and highly readable book, *Every Second Child*, Dr. Archie Kalokerinos describes how he found that by giving infants vitamin C *before* they were immunized, SIDS (Sudden Infant Death Syndrome) could be eliminated. The title refers to the fact that as many as 50 percent of the infants in some aboriginal communities in Australia died, usually of SIDS.[26]

"Have you taken an antioxident today?" pharmacist and nutritionist Earl Mindell asks. He points out that vitamins are our first line of defense against toxic substances. The antioxidents—vitamins A, C, and E and the mineral, selenium—are particularly effective.[27]

"The Last Epidemic"

Currently the epidemic near the top of our list of concerns is one that has been called "The Last Epidemic." This is the poisoning from radioactive fallout following a nuclear war or nuclear power plant accident. As with most projections into the future, the assumption is that everyone will be equally or indiscriminately affected. In the case of radioactive poisoning, the only variable would be distance from the blast or protection by some physical shielding agent.

The radiation sickness and disfiguration that affected the survivors of Hiroshima and Nagasaki are legend, but what is not so well known is that not everyone who was exposed to the radiation suffered radiation poisoning. Some who were only a mile from the center of the blast suffered no ill effects.

At St. Francis Hospital in Nagasaki, which was only a mile from the center of the blast, the entire staff suffered no ill effects. The day after the blast, members of the staff went around the city of Nagasaki to visit and care for the sick in their homes, and in the very part of the city that the Americans had declared would be uninhabitable for the next twenty years! How did they escape? For some time prior to the blast, Dr. Akizuki, one of the directors of the hospital had prepared himself and his co-workers by confining their diet to "yang" foods, in this case, miso soup, brown rice, wakame (seaweed), and Hokkaido

pumpkin. The strict macrobiotic diet they had lived on apparently protected them. According to macrobiotic theory, nuclear radiation is extremely "yin"; therefore, an extremely "yang" diet is needed to
counterbalance it.

Stories of people who recovered from radiation sickness by adopting the macrobiotic diet are sometimes dramatic. A fifty-year-old woman
in Hiroshima who was near the center of the blast and whose body was
burned and penetrated by about 50 glass fragments, recovered by following a strict macrobiotic diet. For one year after the blast she had a
continuous discharge of very black blood from her uterus. Gradually
new blood formed and all the pieces of glass, which were deeply imbed-
ded in her body, came to the surface and were removed one by one.
At the time her story was written (1979) she was in excellent health.[28]

Later researchers have found other nutritional aids helpful in as-
sisting the body to neutralize the harmful effects of radiation. Some of
these are as follows: natural iodine—particularly that found in seaweeds
such as kelp; algin also found in kelp; calcium; vitamin B[6]; the B complex
as found in Brewer's yeast and liver; vitamin C, including the bioflavinoids and rutin; protein; pectin as found in sunflower seeds; and pure,
nonfluoridated water.[29] Vitamin E has been effective in protecting
people from X-ray burns and scarring when taken internally and applied
to the surface *before* exposure.[30] In fact, all the remedies discussed are
most effective taken before exposure and could be called preventive
medicine. Also, with this kind of preventive medicine, we could say
that what will prevent will also cure.

The Latest "Epidemic" (AIDS)

Faith, love, humor, creative visualization, and moral support from a
partner were crucial "medicines" in the recovery of at least one person
from a fatal illness, an illness that has assumed almost panic, if not
epidemic proportions recently. I am referring to AIDS (Auto Immune
Deficiency Syndrome). The patient is William Calderon, who was featured on the cover of *New Realities* (March/April 1985). Along with
mental and emotional support, Calderon followed an optimal nutritional
program that included megadoses of vitamin C, B[12], calcium, vitamin
E, and concentrated vegetable capsules.[31]

As with other "epidemics" only a small percentage of people exposed to the disease actually come down with it; in the case of AIDS
it is 1 to 3 percent.[32] What is the critical factor? Again it is life-style, a
life-style that promotes biochemical imbalances. The immune deficiency
leading to AIDS coincides with the use of drugs, alcohol, and junk foods

(particularly foods high in sugar)—all of which stress the immune system.[33]

Dr. Russell Jaffe, pathologist and toxicologist from the National Institute of Health, ran a series of tests with AIDS patients. The 18 patients who followed Dr. Jaffe's program have been in remission for two and a half years. The program included good health habits with an emphasis on good nutrition plus lots of garlic, vitamins, minerals, intravenous vitamin C, ginseng for low energy, procaine, and plenty of sleep and exercise. Since many patients had amoebas and other parasites in their colon, they were given a drug (flagyl) to kill the parasites.* Many had yeast, fungus, and candida albicans, so they were given nystatin and put on a low fungus diet.[34] Al Battista, N.D., feels that candida is a precursor to AIDS; AIDS being the final breakdown of the immune system when candida gets out of control. How do people get candida albicans? Again, it is the result of practices that unbalance internal ecology or biochemistry. In this case, they include the taking of antibiotics, steroids, and birth control pills.[35]

What other unbalancing factors in our environment or life-style could suppress immune function? "Has the possibility of a connection between AIDS, cancer and the chemical age been explored?" Isabel Jansen, R.N., asks. AIDS is a 20th-century disease, she points out, and we need to look at our 20th-century environment for the cause rather than at practices such as homosexuality and prostitution which have been with us for centuries.[36]

Many chemicals in our environment are known immune suppressors, e.g., lead and mercury, but the most widely used and abused is probably fluoride. Besides inhibiting or destroying enzymes, fluoride damages white blood cells and their chromosomes, and interferes with DNA function—all such processes weaken the immune system. In comparing four cities, Isabel Jansen found three times as many AIDS cases (per million population) in cities where the water was fluoridated as in those where it was not.**

One of the more significant contributions to our understanding of AIDS is described in *AIDS: The Mystery and the Solution* by Alan Cantwell Jr., M.D.[37] His research suggests that AIDS is associated with immunosuppressive factors such as: (1) poverty and its attendant mal-

---

*A more "whole" approach, of course, would be to get rid of the waste material that feeds the parasites.
**Earlier studies in the United States and Canada have shown cancer death rates 4 to 40 percent higher in areas where the water is fluoridated than in areas where it is not. (John Yiamouyiannis, Ph.D., *Fluoride The Aging Factor*, Health Action Press, Delaware, Ohio, 1983)

nutrition, overcrowding, and lack of sanitation; (2) immunosuppressive diseases such as tuberculosis, leprosy, and "opportunistic" (yeast, fungus, or parasite) infections; (3) the use of immunosuppressive drugs such as those used in antibiotic therapy and chemotherapy; (4) radiation therapy; and (5) drug abuse.

AIDS is a form of cancer, according to Cantwell, caused by similar-appearing acid-fast bacteria which are found in the affected tissues of both diseases. However, these same bacteria, which Cantwell calls the "cancer microbe," are found within the blood and tissues of all human beings, both healthy and sick, as well as in animals. The AIDS virus, HTLV-3, isolated in 1984 by government scientists was found in 88 percent of a group of American patients. Again, however, the virus antibody is found in some AIDS patients and not in others. (The HTLV-3 blood test does not detect the presence of live virus, only antibodies to the virus.) In fact, the vast majority of people who tested positive for AIDS antibodies were perfectly healthy.

The AIDS virus, like the cancer microbe, is highly pleomorphic, so much so that making a vaccine would be difficult if not impossible. Cantwell quotes a couple of researchers who think that some viruses may be either part of the life cycle or a deficient form of a bacterium. (He discusses the work of other researchers who describe "a specific life cycle" of the cancer organism very much like the work of Rife and others discussed in Chapter 5.)

Where do immunizations fit into this picture? The AIDS HTLV-3 virus is an RNA retrovirus. These viruses are equipped with a special enzyme, reverse transcriptase, which allows them to form strands of DNA, thus enabling them to become integrated with the DNA of the cells they infect.* It is this integration within the chromosomal material of the cell which changes the cell and can cause it to become malignant. (See discussion of viruses in Chapters 2 and 5.) The immune process cannot act against the virus because it no longer exists as a virus, but as a particle of nucleic acid hidden within the chromosomal material of the cell. Live viruses, the primary antigenic material of vaccines, can, as we learned earlier, seed the body with "molecules in search of a disease," which under conducive conditions can become activated and cause degenerative diseases such as cancer/AIDS.

Does all this sound familiar? Why do statistics at the Centers for Disease Control (CDC) continue to show that homosexual or bisexual men are most at risk, when evidence is coming from Africa and other

---

*Viruses without this enzyme can also integrate their genetic material into the genetic material of human and animal cells. Viruses with the reverse transcriptase enzyme, however, have been specifically implicated in cancer.

places that AIDS is predominantly a heterosexual disease associated with poverty and many of the immunosuppressive practices of Modern Medicine? Here, according to Cantwell, are some of the ways statistics are managed to create this impression: (1) listing homosexual intravenous drug addicts in the homosexual-bisexual risk group rather than in the drug abuse group. (2) Excluding patients from being diagnosed as having AIDS if they are either over 60 and have Kaposi's sarcoma, or if they are patients who have been on immunosuppressive drugs for treatment of cancer and other diseases, (3) Diagnosing AIDS with certainty if opportunistic infection and/or Kaposi's sarcoma appear in high-risk patients, i.e., male homosexuals, intravenous drug abusers, Haitian refugees, hemophiliacs, infants receiving blood transfusions, female sexual partners of males with AIDS, male prison inmates, and female prostitutes.

Are we seeing what we want to see, creating melodramas that appeal to some perverse need for sexploitation? If AIDS is "Falwell's revenge" for our sexual sins, why does just a relatively small percentage of female prostitutes contract it, the majority of whom are drug abusers?

The power of conditioned response, the tendency to interpret data in terms congenial to our educational and cultural conditioning as well as to our emotional and ego needs, is illustrated by Cantwell's interpretation of his data. How can he, I asked myself, an internationally known researcher in the field of cancer microbiology, say positively that the cancer microbe causes AIDS when the AIDS/cancer microbe resides within all of us? He speaks of the omnipresence of bacteria in our bodies, which probably help us to maintain our health, and how these same bacteria can become dangerous and pathogenic when the immune system becomes damaged or weakened. The obvious cause of AIDS is a weakened or damaged immune system, not a particular bacteria. Why doesn't medical research focus on what factors in our environment and in our lives weaken the immune system? Is this too simple? too ordinary? too undramatic? Or does it threaten too many vested interests, and isn't it easier to get publicity and money for research when white-coated heroes are stalking an enemy—a mysterious, microscopic enemy?

The Immunization Connection

"In a flash, I knew I had solved not only the riddle of AIDS, but also of the dramatic increase in the cases of childhood leukemia, birth defects, and other malignancies and many chronic, degenerative conditions." So wrote Eva Lee Snead, M.D., as she was describing her breakthrough research in a cover story in *Health Freedom News* of July 1987 entitled "AIDS—Immunization Related Syndrome."

Dr. Snead was researching the SV-40 virus because of its similarity to HIV, the final name given to the AIDS virus. (The AIDS virus has received several names.) SV-40 virus is a powerful immunosuppressor and activator of HIV. It causes a clinical syndrome indistinguishable from AIDS as well as birth defects, leukemia, and other malignancies. How does one acquire SV-40? As far as we know, it can only be acquired by direct contact with or eating the meat of its natural carrier, the African green monkey.

Who would eat green monkey soup? But, Dr. Snead asks, "What if the green monkey soup had been stained pink and served on a sugar cube?"

To learn more about the African monkey, Dr. Snead went to the medical library to begin her research. After noticing the "incredible amount of references (392 in the 'Medline system' since 1980 alone) to this ape" she became familiar with and puzzled by the expression SV-40, or Simian Virus-40, constantly associated with the African green monkey. Combing through the Index Medicus catalogs, year by year, she noticed a strange phenomenon: All references listed under the name SV-40 stopped abruptly in 1964. She decided to look under the word "monkey." "Ten minutes later I had more information than I wanted to find, and fate placed a monkey on my back that I wished I had never encountered. . . . What had I come across? In front of my eyes was the following citation:

"Excretion of SV-40 virus after oral administration of *contaminated polio vaccine*, [italics mine] Horvath, B. L., and Fornosi F., *Acta Microbiologica Scientaria Hungary*, Vol. 11:271–75, 1964–65."

This was the breakthrough for Dr. Snead. Though her continued research was laborious, it was fascinating. Unlike most research projects where increased information frequently casts doubt on the original hypothesis and therefore the validity of the conclusions, her research showed only increased promise and affirmation. She became convinced that the cause of AIDS and the other diseases mentioned was SV-40 contamination of some batches of immunizations.

Over 30 years ago I remember reading "horror" stories of the slaughter of thousands of monkeys to make Salk vaccine and now I was reading of "a recently discovered virus, unwittingly put into hundreds of thousands, if not millions, of doses of early Salk vaccine." The unknown virus is, of course, SV-40 and the publication is *Science Digest*, 1963. Arthur J. Snider, the author of the article, "Near Disaster with the Salk Vaccine," downplays the seriousness of the situation, but I couldn't help thinking as I read Dr. Snead's article, "If AIDS isn't Falwell's revenge, could it be the monkey's revenge?"

Before leaving Dr. Snead and going on to another substantiating event, some quotations from various professional journals cited in her article are worth noting: "Scientific data have been reviewed which show that the problem of the oncogenic [tumor causing] potential of live virus vaccines should be regarded as an urgent one." "It appears from what has been said that infectious disease and malnutrition are so inextricably interwoven with each other that any attempt to deal with them separately . . . is as futile as trying to separate the effects of heredity and environment." And finally an article from "Public Health Reports" (Vol. 77, No. 2, Feb. 1962) titled "Survey of Childhood Malignancies" points out that "children between ages 2 and 4 years of age have been more affected by the unfavorable trend of leukemia mortality than any other age group under 70 years." Particularly ironic was the statement that "the recent increase in leukemia deaths happened sooner in technically advanced countries" and that the determining factor was not affluence but "the availability of medical services."

The detrimental effect of "the availability of medical services" was recently dramatized by a front-page article in *The Times* of London, May 11, 1987: "Smallpox vaccine 'triggered Aids virus.' " An advisor to the World Health Organization (WHO), the organization which masterminded the 13-year vaccination campaign which ended in 1980, told *The Times*: "I thought it was just a coincidence until we studied the latest findings about the reactions which can be caused by *Vaccinia* [smallpox vaccine]. Now I believe the smallpox vaccine theory is the explanation to the explosion of Aids."

The smallpox vaccine theory accounts for a number of phenomena: (1) The seven central African states most affected are the same states where the most intensive immunization programs were carried out. (2) Brazil, the only South American country covered in the immunization campaign, had the highest incidence of AIDS in that region. (3) There is less sign of infection among 5 to 11 year olds in Central Africa. (4) AIDS is associated with homosexuality in the West, whereas in Africa it is spread more evenly among males and females. Explanation: About 14,000 Haitians who were with the United Nations armed services in Africa were covered in the immunization program. They returned home when Haiti had become a popular playground for San Francisco homosexuals. (5) The AIDS organism previously regarded by scientists as "weak, slow and vulnerable" began to behave with the strength capable of creating a plague. Explanation: The use of live virus vaccines, like that used for smallpox, can activate dormant virus infections such as the human immunodeficiency virus (HIV) associated with AIDS.

Because this theory would be devastating not only to the WHO but to other public health campaigns for immunizations as well as the continued use of smallpox vaccine in AIDS research, many experts are reluctant to support it. *The Times* mollifies its readers by pointing out that the 13-year smallpox eradication campaign saved two million lives a year and 15 million infections with a global saving of $1,000 million a year. Where these figures come from is anyone's guess.

The Mind Connection

Our discussion of the relationship between holism and epidemics would be incomplete without once again underscoring the pivotal role of the mind. A number of scientists have said that what we call reality is perceptual agreement; that is, consensual reality. One of the more bizarre epidemics of history illustrates the point which is, to paraphrase Rupert Sheldrake, that much of what we consider truth, or "laws of nature," may be only habits of perception. Our knowledge is part of our culture; we see and look for what we know.

A strange malady occurred during the Middle Ages in the southeastern part of Italy known as Apulia. "People, asleep or awake, would suddenly jump up, feeling an acute pain like the sting of a bee. Some saw the spider, others did not, but they knew that it must be the tarantula. They ran out of the house into the street, to the market place dancing in great excitement. Soon they were joined by others who like them had just been bitten, or by people who had been stung in previous years, for the disease was never quite cured. The poison remained in the body and was reactivated every year by the heat of summer. People were known to have relapsed every summer for thirty years."[38] "Music and dancing were the only effective remedies, and people were known to have died within an hour or in a few days because music was not available. A member of Dr. Ferdinandus' own family, his cousin, Francesco Franco, died thus within twenty-four hours because no musician could be found after he had been stung."[39] "After having thus danced for a number of days, the people were exhausted—and cured, at least for the time being. But they knew that the poison was in them and that every summer the tunes of the tarantella would revive their frenzy."[40]

Though the malady reportedly continued for several centuries, it wasn't until the 17th century that the disease was studied and recorded. The physicians of the day accepted the popular theory that the disease was due to the bite of the tarantula; however, when these same tarantulas were shipped to other parts of the country they seemed to lose their venom. The spider was venomous in Apulia only. According to one report, a wasp, a rooster, and even the tarantula herself danced whenever she heard the music. However, this phenomenon occurred only in Apulia.

According to another report, a skeptical physician in Naples had himself bitten in the left arm by two Apulian tarantulas in August 1693 before six witnesses and a public notary. The arm became somewhat swollen, but otherwise he felt no ill effects. People rationalized that it was the scorching heat of Apulia that activated the virus and gave it its specific effect; but again, in other countries just as hot as Apulia where the same tarantula occurred, there was no such thing as tarantism (the name given the malady).

The doctors tried the usual treatments of the day: scarifying the wound with a lancet or cauterizing it with a red hot iron; however, the great majority of patients had no wound. Internally the doctors gave antidotes such as treacle or brandy. Finally, the doctors had to admit there was no cure except music, not any music, but only the tunes played in Apulia for centuries as the treatment for tarantism. They theorized that the dances created by the music caused the patients to perspire, thereby driving out the poison and curing them—at least for the season. Sometime during the middle of the 18th century the disease died out.[41]

What could have caused this strange malady? The historian Epiphanius Ferdinandus gives us a clue. "He said that according to some people tarantism was not a disease at all, a view that he refuted immediately with the argument that if tarantism was a mere fiction, there would not be so many poor people, and particularly women, spending nearly all their money on the music." Henry Sigerist, medical doctor and historian, apparently unravels the mystery when he suggests that tarantism was a nervous disorder, a kind of neurosis brought about by conflict between the beliefs and customs of the Greek tradition, which had been strong in Apulia, with the new Christianity that inundated the old culture. The old deities such as Dionysus, Cybele, and Demeter, and the orgiastic rites that were part of their worship, were buried; but the primitive instincts and the need to express the emotions associated with them did not disappear. Instead they became legitimatized in the form of dancing as victims of tarantism. (The similarity of these rites to the symptoms of tarantism is striking.)

The power of the mind and emotions to create and correct disease states has been widely discussed. "Every thought you have creates changes in the body," according to Norman Shealy, M.D. He says that joy increases the strength of the immune system and sadness or depression decreases the strength of the immune system.* He illustrates his point by telling stories of people who, by following a meditation-visualization program, recovered from often serious and incapacitating illnesses. (Counseling, autogenic training and good nutrition were also part of his program.)[42]

"We use hypnosis like a surgeon uses his scalpel. We cut into a person's psyche to find the root cause of his physical disease. Then we remove it . . . curing the disease," Dr. Pavel Bul, therapist at Leningrad's Pavlov Medical Institute, revealed. He said his studies show conclusively that almost all cases of asthma, allergy, and hypertension have strong emotional roots.[43]

If mind and not matter is primary and if we are all connected in some transpersonal sense, then transfer of mental and emotional states, sometimes called "psychic contagion," can occur.

In March 1982, I heard on the news that in the previous year Norfolk Catholic High School in Virginia had experienced an epidemic. At first it had been called the flu; then doctors suspected carbon monoxide poisoning; and, finally, an epidemiologist in the area said the disease was psycho-social. People "caught" the disease by seeing their friends get it.

If the thought patterns in our mind affect the thought patterns of all other minds, could consensual reality be thought of as a contagion or confluence of mental images? Quantum theory reveals that we live in an ocean of force fields, that fields generate objects, and that an object is simply a highly concentrated aspect of a field—thought (the field) structures matter (the body). The mind and the images of reality it holds are the pivot upon which the destiny of the body turns; the images of many minds can be the pivot upon which the destiny of a group or even the world turns.

Robert Ingersoll once remarked that had he been God he would have made health contagious instead of disease. "When shall we come to recognize that health is as contagious as disease," an Indian contemporary responded. Virtue is as contagious as vice and cheerfulness is as contagious as moroseness, he continued.[44] When the mental images of a community of minds are filled with pictures of health rather than disease, the possibilities for the realization of health become practically

*Negative emotions trigger the release of norepinephrine, an immune suppressor. ("Psychoimmunology: for each state of mind, a state of body?" *Brain/Mind Bulletin*, Dec. 10, 1984, p. 3.) Also, Larry Dossey, M.D., points out that "thought and emotion affect the immune system at cellular and subcellular levels." (*Brain/Mind Bulletin*, July 29, 1985, p. 2.)

limitless. This interconnectedness and blurring of boundaries is beautifully expressed by Dr. Larry Dossey: "Isolated derangements at the level of the atoms simply do not occur. All information is everywhere transmitted. Crisp, causal events that were once thought to characterize each and every human disease fade into endless reverberating chains of happenings. . . . We see the molecular theory of disease causation as an outmoded, picturesque description. Discrete causes never occur in individual bodies for the simple reason that discrete individual bodies do not themselves exist." Dr. Dossey refers to the "space-time" model of health in which the body is not regarded as an object surrounded by empty space, but as a pattern and process whose boundaries are "always fading, reforming, and fading again in the endless round of biodance." Because of the "profound interrelations between consciousness and the physical world: we should strive to maximize rather than minimize the subjective element in the healing process, he points out. Purposeful change can be initiated by patients as well as professional healers. "Each patient has the potential of being his own healer. Healing becomes democratized."[45]

NOTES

1. Lewis Thomas, *The Lives of a Cell*, Bantam Books, New York, 1974, p. 6.
2. From a flier announcing a conference to be given at the New York Academy of Medicine on the subject, "Mind and Immunity," April 1982.
3. "Psychoimmunology: for each state of mind, a state of body?" *Brain/Mind Bulletin*, Dec. 10, 1984.
4. Marcus Bach, "Holistic Healing," lecture at A.R.E., Virginia Beach, Va., Dec. 29, 1976.
5. Ibid.
6. "Spanish Flu of 1918 Worst Killer of All," (UPI), Los Angeles Times, Jan. 12, 1969, pp. 7–8.
7. Ibid.
8. Henry Sigerist, *Civilization and Disease*, Cornell University Press, 1943, p. 236. Dr. Sigerist gives the figure of 10 million lives lost to the influenza epidemic of 1918–19. Ms. Hume gives the figure of 8 million lives lost, excluding China, Japan, South America, and great tracts of Asia and Africa. (Ethyl Douglas Hume, *Bechamp or Pasteur?*, The C. W. Daniel Co, Ltd., Saffron Walden, Essex, England, p. 220.)

9. Hume, *Bechamp or Pasteur?*, pp. 220–26. Also, R. B. Pearson, *Fasting and Man's Correct Diet*, Health Research, Mokelumne Hill, Calif., 1921, pp. 136–39.
10. "How One Doctor Cured the 1918 Flu," *Organic Consumer Report*, Oct. 5, 1976.
11. Thomas, op. cit., pp. 6–7.
12. Christopher Bird, "What has become of the Rife Microscope?" *New Age Journal*, Jan. 26, 1976, p. 42.
13. Royal E. S. Hays, M.D., "The Germ Theory," *The Homeopathic Review*, May 1947, reprinted by Nell and Guy Rogers, *The Medical Mischief, You Say!*, Health Research, Pasadena, Calif., 1953, p. 35.
14. William Dufty quoting William Coda Martin, M.D., *Sugar Blues*, Warner Books, New York, 1975, p. 154.
15. "Spanish Flu of 1918 Worst Killer of All," op. cit.
16. Leonard Wickenden, *Our Daily Poison*, Hillman Books, New York, 1961, p. 57.
17. Ibid.
18. "Are You Getting Too Much Fluoride?", *Better Nutrition*, Dec. 1981, p. 49.
19. From a flier from Eden Ranch, publishers of Organic Consumer Report, undated (probably published in the early 1960s).
20. Morton Biskind, M.D., "Public Health Aspects of the New Insecticides," *American Journal of Digestive Diseases*, Nov. 1953, p. 333.
21. Ibid. p. 338.
22. Ibid. p. 338 (note).
23. Ibid. p. 338.
24. Paavo Airola, N.D., Ph.D., *Every Woman's Book*, Health Plus, Phoenix, Ariz., 1979, p. 290. (Dr. Airola gives us six scientific references as a sample.)
25. Archie Kalokerinos, M.D., *Every Second Child*, Keats Publishing, 1981.
26. Airola, op. cit., p. 290.
27. Earl Mindell, *Vitamin Bible*, Warner Books, New York, 1979.
28. Leonard Jacobs, "Natural Ways to Survive a Meltdown," *East/West Journal*, June 1979, p. 66.
29. Linda Clark, *Stay Young Longer*, Pyramid Books, New York, 1971, p. 117. Also Linda Clark, *Linda Clark's Handbook of Natural Remedies for Common Ailments*, Pocket Books, New York, 1977, p. 176.
30. Adelle Davis, *Let's Get Well*, Harcourt, Brace, & World, New York, 1965, p. 381.

31. Jean Shinoda Bolen, M.D., "William Calderon's Triumph Over AIDS Brings New Hope," *New Realities*, March/April 1985, pp. 9–15.
32. Larry Eppolito, Assistant Director of AIDS Clinic in Los Angeles, Donahue Show, Sept. 20, 1985.
33. Maureen Salaman, "Dr. Michael Gerber on Aids and Prevention," *Health Freedom News*, Sept. 1985, as Maureen interviews Dr. Gerber, p. 9.
34. Michael Gerber, M.D., ibid.
35. Al Battista, N.D., "Candida Albicans, Maureen Salaman interviews Al Battista," *Health Freedom News*, Nov. 1984, p. 25.
36. Isabel Jansen, R.N., "Aids and the Chemical Age," *Health Freedom News*, Sept. 1986, pp. 16–17.
37. Alan Cantwell, Jr., M.D., *Aids: The Mystery and the Solution*, Aries Rising Press, Los Angeles, Calif., 1986.
38. Henry E. Sigerist, *Civilization and Disease*, Cornell University Press, Ithaca, N.Y., 1943, p. 218.
39. Ibid., p. 219.
40. Ibid., p. 221.
41. Ibid., p. 224.
42. Norman Shealy, M.D., "Autogenic Training," Association for Research and Enlightenment, Virginia Beach, Va., Aug. 30, 1977.
43. *Organic Consumer Report*, "Organic Seeds for Thought," Sept. 28, 1982.
44. Huston Smith, *The Religions of Man*, Harper and Row, New York, 1965, p. 117.
45. Larry Dossey, M.D., "Space, Time, and Medicine," *ReVision*, Fall 1982, pp. 54–55.

SUGGESTED ADDITIONAL READING

Harvey Diamond and Marilyn Diamond, *Living Health*, Warner Books, New York, 1987.
Michael A. Weiner, Ph.D., *Maximum Immunity*, Houghton Mifflin, Boston, 1986.

8

■

"BEAUTIFUL" AND "UGLY" SOLUTIONS

Anything which is forced or misunderstood can never be beautiful.

XENOPHON

THE "BEAUTIFUL" SOLUTION

The Aesthetic Criterion

"Beauty is truth, truth beauty," wrote the poet John Keats over 150 years ago in his "Ode to a Grecian Urn." Now, 20th-century scientists are telling us that beauty is a means of discovering truth as well as a standard by which it is recognized. In science you can recognize truth by its beauty and simplicity, physicist Richard Feynman points out. "Werner Heisenberg declared that beauty 'in exact science, no less than in the arts, is the most important source of illumination and clarity.' "[1] As a standard in physics beauty even takes primacy over experiment.

The three elements of beauty specified by physicists are simplicity, harmony, and brilliance. Contained within the principle of simplicity are completeness and economy; contained within the principle of harmony is symmetry; and contained within the principle of brilliance are clarity and resonance, or the ability to shed light on other phenomena.[2]

"A beautiful solution or proof is one that is simple, direct, that goes to the very nature and essence of the problem. An ugly one, though perfectly correct and usable somehow misses this essence."[3] John Holt refers here to mathematics, paraphrasing a point made by Wertheimer in his book, *Productive Thinking.* Can we apply this standard, as well as the standard of beauty specified by physicists, to the fields of health care?

Let's begin by asking the obvious: Does the practice of immunizing people—or searching for a vaccine—for every identifiable disease go "to the very nature and essence of the problem"? Is this solution the simple and direct one? Is it conducive to a sense of harmony within oneself and with the natural world? Is it economical, not only in terms of money but of time and energy expenditure?

Since immunization programs are central to the existence of public health departments, the practice of pediatrics, and much public funded research, we might ask these questions of our entire health care system. Let's apply to the health care system our three criteria of beauty: simplicity, harmony, and brilliance.

Simplicity. A beautiful health care system would be based on theories that are simple without being simplistic. The fundamental ideas could be understood and applied by most people. The theories would be economical; that is, they would explain a wide range of phenomena in the simplest, easiest, most direct way possible. The theories would be complete in that they would be logical and consistent. In practice the program would be economical, not only in terms of money, but in terms of time and energy expenditure.

Harmony. A beautiful theory of health would promote a sense of harmony with the natural world. It would perceive other life forms as intelligent, responsive, and life supporting; our relations with them would be dependent upon our own actions and perceptions. We now know, for instance, that even microorganisms show signs of intelligence as well as responsiveness to human thought and emotion.[4]

The principle of harmony is implied in the idea of holism. If we think of a disease process as part of a larger process or whole, we know that a part cannot be altered without altering the whole. This suggests that any action directed to a part must be harmonized with the welfare of the whole. For instance, a holistic doctor would know that a treatment to prevent or correct a disease would change the body-mind, not only in relation to the disease being treated, but in relation to other diseases as well. Therefore, his treatments would be directed toward enhancing the life of the body as a whole as well as the life of the person as a whole.

The elegance of balanced proportions is suggested by the principle of symmetry. It is suggested not only anatomically—e.g., duality and complementarity of right and left sides of our bodies—but in the idea of balancing our lives. As we discussed earlier, life-style and "think-style" are primary determinants of health or its lack.

Brilliance. Implied in the above discussion.

An elegantly simple and harmonious health care system would be conducive to personal growth and empowerment. Therefore, its theories and practices would be directed towards personal autonomy; creative and egalitarian interaction with others, including health care professionals; and the promotion of a sense of harmony and relatedness to one's own body-mind as well as the natural world. It would focus on the characteristics of health rather than the characteristics of disease, promoting the former rather than fighting or avoiding the latter. It would be oriented toward correcting causes rather than treating symptoms; therefore, it would encourage long-term rather than short-term or quick fix solutions; for, like great works of art, beautiful solutions stand the test of time.

Are there any health care systems or schools of healing that have most of the above characteristics? Generally speaking, any of the "natural"* schools of healing will promote personal autonomy and independence, nonauthoritarian ways of relating to health care professionals, and a sense of harmony and relatedness to one's own body-mind as well as the natural world. These schools of healing are called natural, not so much because they generally make minimal use of technological intervention, but because they work directly with the natural healing energies of the body and the natural world.

Natural therapies generally assume a life or mind principle—variously referred to as the "vital force," the "innate," "ch'i"—that sustains and heals the body-mind. Central to the philosophy of natural healing is the idea that the body is self-healing and that the purpose of a therapeutic modality should be to arouse and support this healing energy.

Energy and Natural Healing

"I sing the body electric," said the poet Walt Whitman. "The body is electrical in nature," William McGarey, M.D., told his audience. "The medicine of the future will be electrical in nature."[5]

---

*Natural in this context means using no toxic substances such as drugs and vaccines and no invasive procedures such as surgery.

Understanding and treating the body as energy rather than mass is an idea as old as civilization. Forty-five centuries ago, a Chinese physician named Koai Yu Chu identified the unity of matter and energy and described a "primordial energy that gives birth to all the elements and is integrated into them." This energy, which the Chinese later called *Ch'i*, is the life force of the universe as well as the healing and sustaining energy of the body.[6] When this energy is blocked, illness results. The purpose of the healer is to release the blockage so the energy can flow freely. This is the theory behind acupuncture and acupressure, of course. If we think of healing as balancing as well as restoring the energy within the body, we can include such health care systems as macrobiotics, chiropractic, homeopathy, naturopathy, and herbology.

In general, natural schools of healing such as these, avoid the use of toxic substances such as drugs and vaccines, because they interfere in subtle ways with the free flow of this energy, or vital force. Any toxic substance, whether exogenous (originating outside the body) or endogenous (originating inside the body) is part of the problem, not the solution. Also, natural schools of healing generally interpret disease symptoms as part of a healing process, not as an enemy to be fought, so a toxic system of weaponry would have no place.

A number of writers have mistakenly identified the principle of vaccination with the principle of the law of similars in homeopathy. The law of similars asserts that, "Like will be cured by like—a like remedy in minimum dose." In other words, the substance that produces the same symptoms in a healthy person as in a sick person, if given in sufficiently small doses, will cure the illness.* The differences between the application of this principle and the principle behind vaccination are major:

(1) The homeopathic dose is much smaller than that used in vaccines; in fact, the homeopathic medicine is diluted to the point where there is no trace of the original substance—only an energy pattern. (This is achieved by a process known as "potentization" in which the dynamic energy latent in a substance is liberated by a succession of dilutions and mechanical agitation.) So the homeopathic dose is essentially an energy therapy designed to arouse and strengthen the natural healing energy, or vital force, of the body. It is not directed at microorganisms or their destruction, but to the patient and the strengthening of his vital forces.

(2) The homeopathic remedy is holistic; it addresses the uniqueness

---

*This makes sense only when we abandon the adversarial view of disease and see its symptoms as part of a larger healing process.

of the patient as well as his wholeness. The patient as a mental and spiritual being is studied and treated as well as the patient as a physical organism. Herd treatment and prescriptions, such as those prescribed by compulsory immunization laws, would be contrary to the homeopathic philosophy and ideals.

(3) Homeopathic remedies are not made from disease products or agents, that is, viruses or bacteria, but from simple, raw substances: mineral, vegetable, or animal.

(4) Homeopaths generally do not use injections. It is contrary to the homeopathic philosophy "to violate the integrity of the body by forcibly introducing medicinal agents by other than the natural orifices and channels."[7]

Homeopaths can use oral immunizing agents, however. Certain of these highly attenuated, harmless preparations can be used as immunizing agents for most transmittable diseases as well as to counteract the undesirable side effects of conventional immunization antigens.

A sense of harmony, relatedness, and personal empowerment is promoted by the philosophy of homeopathy. It assumes a Life or Mind entity that creates and sustains the physical organism. The working principle of this Life or Mind is the Law of Reciprocal Action, otherwise known as the law of balance. It is variously called the law of compensation, rhythm, polarity, vibration, or just action-reaction; and it is operative in the mental and spiritual realms as well as in the physical realm. The expression of Life or Mind is The Law of Love which is always beneficent, creative, and harmonizing. "Hence, the consistent practitioner of homeopathy never uses, and has no need to use, any irritating, weakening, depressing, infecting, intoxicating or injurious agent of any kind in the treatment of the sick."[8]

Perhaps the baseline of all schools of natural healing is naturopathy, or Nature Cure as it is known in England. Its "medicines" are such things as sunshine, fresh air, pure water, natural foods, and regular periods of internal cleansing through juice or water fasts and colonics. Manipulative therapies such as chiropractic and reflexology; nontoxic herbal and homeopathic medicines; and hydrotherapy (the therapeutic uses of water), are also part of the naturopathic "tool kit." Recently, iridology, the science of reading the degree of tissue activity of the various organs of the body by the markings in the iris, has been used by many naturopaths.

Iridology bears out one of the basic premises of naturopathy, namely that disease develops through an orderly progression of increasing toxic encumbrance in the body. All forms of disease are caused by an accumulation of toxins in the system according to naturopathy, and the purpose of any therapeutic program is to assist the body to rid itself of these poisons.

Through iridology we can trace the progression of disease from acute to degenerative, the acute stage being the active discharge stage and the degenerative stage being the stage of tissue destruction. The model works something like this. First, we have a cold or some acute mucous elimination. We take a cold remedy to stop the discharge of mucous. The cold disappears but later—sometimes many years later— bronchitis, flu, boils, cysts, or a running ear develops. Again we take suppressant drugs and the symptoms disappear. Later—again sometimes many years later—we develop hayfever or pneumonia. Years later, after dosing with more shots and drugs, we develop asthma or rheumatism. Finally, after further physiological insult with drugs and shots, we develop degenerative diseases such as cancer, arthritis and gangrene. We have progressed from an acute illness to a subacute one and from there to a chronic, then subchronic, and finally to a degenerative disease.

To cure a disease we have to cleanse the body, so the body can replace degenerative tissue with new. We must retrace the disease process and arrive at the acute stage again wherein the body regains the vitality necessary to throw off what doesn't belong to it. When we take drugs to stop the discharge—a symptom of elimination—we push not only the toxic material but the drugs as well back into the tissues and create "toxic settlements."

One of the pioneers in researching and teaching people the principles of health is the distinguished nutritionist, iridologist, naturopath, and chiropractor, Dr. Bernard Jensen. In his book, *The Science and Practice of Iridology*, he presents case histories illustrating the retracing process. Dr. Jensen told one woman, whose iris showed a great deal of sulfur settlement in the brain area, that she would probably have a sulfur elimination during the course of her therapy. Her gray hair turned completely yellow as the sulfur was eliminated through her scalp. During this elimination crisis she developed diarrhea and remembered when she was a child that her grandmother had given her sulfur and molasses as a spring tonic. In a couple of months after the elimination process, her hair returned to its natural black color.

Another case describes a very thin young man with a stomach ulcer who wanted to know how to gain weight. During the healing crisis he developed a high fever and delirium, a painful headache, and extreme pains in the head around the ears. He then remembered having this same condition one time on a trip to Alaska. Nothing was done for the condition while on the trip except that drugs were administered. During the eliminative process he tasted the same drugs he had taken years before. After the crisis he gained 15 pounds and felt wonderful.

Even mental disturbances can be corrected by a process of cleansing and rebalancing the body. One woman, after trying a number of different schools of healing including medicine and chiropractic, was healed of compulsive and intermittent crying by fasting, living on natural foods, and exercising regularly. During her healing crisis she developed a fever, her crying returned, and her head became infested with lice! In questioning the patient, Dr. Jensen found that when she was a child she had head lice, and kerosene had been used to destroy them. This had suppressed the condition and the lice lay dormant beneath the scalp. The healing crisis caused the crying spells and lice to resurface as part of the retracing process.[9]

Could we say that "sickness is something trying to come out"? Seen in this light sickness is a complement to health. It is the body-mind's attempt to (1) cleanse itself, (2) heal itself, (3) rebalance itself, and (4) teach us. From Hippocrates, who saw the primary function of disease as the body's attempt to re-establish harmony within itself, to Freud, who saw the healing of the psyche as resulting primarily from the discharge of negative emotions that were locked into painful experiences in the past, the theme of purging and rebalancing in healing is perennial. We might call this The Healing Archetype.*

What about childhood diseases? Why do children seem to be more susceptible to colds and runny noses than adults? The conventional explanation of this susceptibility is that their immune systems are immature, and they haven't built sufficient resistance to the "bugs going around." Quite the contrary, Dr. Jensen maintains. Because children usually have more runny noses and colds than the adults with whom they live indicates their bodies are vital enough to throw off toxic material; whereas adults, whose bodies are generally less vital and more encumbered, tend to store toxic materials. The capacity for acute illness, either the initial illness or a healing crisis, indicates a comparatively high level of energy and physical vitality. Childhood diseases are really a subacute form of disease, the initial cold or runny nose being the acute form that was suppressed by drugs or other unnatural substances.

It has been said, usually pejoratively, that naturopaths don't believe in germs or immunizations. Certainly immunizations would be contrary to the naturopathic philosophy. Dr. Jensen, for instance, devotes over two pages of his book, *You Can Master Disease*, to the destructive

---

*This idea was perverted by the medical profession into practices of bloodletting, violent purging, and leeches and cupping.

effects of immunizations. He quotes a number of eminent medical doctors and studies that point to a link between childhood immunizations and the later appearance of polio, meningitis, and cancer. "Artificial immunizations and drugs injure the nerves, the cerebral cortex, the heart, the kidneys, and the glands, and chronic disease is the result," Dr. Jensen states.[10]

Naturopaths do not believe in the medical interpretation of germs. They maintain that bacteria (germs) are created by dead and decaying tissue. Their function is a cleansing one—to feed upon toxic material until it is gone; hence, the naturopathic emphasis on keeping the body clean. Dr. John Christopher, an outstanding herbalist and naturopathic doctor, encouraged fevers in his patients so the germs could do their work better!*

Recent Research

Recent research bears out many of the premises of natural healing. The idea, for instance, that disease results from energy blockage has been corroborated by the researches of Dr. Otto Warburg, two-time Nobel prizewinner in Cellular Physiology and Medicine, and Dr. William Frederick Koch, whom I discussed in Chapter 4. Energy production on the cellular level, they have found, is the key to health or disease. This energy production is the same as the cell respiration referred to in Chapter 4 as the oxidation process. The blocking of this process is "the most important cause of malignant, viral, bacterial and allergic diseases," they point out. "Effective prevention and treatment of these diseases depends upon the restoration and maintenance of the normal oxidation process." Dr. Koch also proved that "blocked oxidation in microorganisms causes them to be pathogenic and parasitic, and that when this condition [is] corrected these organisms become non-pathogenic, non-parasitic and non-virulent."[11] Oxygen deficiency and the presence of certain toxic substances block the oxidation process in the body. To restore health the following modalities are used: (1) an oxidation catalyst in conjunction with colonics: (2) organically grown food—food grown without toxic fertilizers and pesticides—eaten mostly raw; and (3) chelated minerals.[12]

---

*An interesting experiment with lizards demonstrates the importance of the cleansing function of fevers. Lizards were injected with potentially fatal doses of bacteria. When the lizards crawled under a heat lamp which raised their body temperature 3 degrees, 75 percent of them survived. When no heat was available, the lizards couldn't raise their body temperature, and 75 percent of them died. (Ronald Kotulak, "Desert lizards led researcher to theory that fever may help body fight disease," *Miami Herald*, reprinted by *Health Science*, April/May 1981.)

A simple illustration of the pleomorphic nature of microorganisms can be found in the bacteria of the human intestine. Healthy intestinal bacteria manufacture many nutrients, including vitamins B and K, and "strongly influence the internal balance of cholesterol and biliary compounds (digestive juices) made from it." Miles Robinson, M.D., goes on to say that "it is important that the intestinal bacteria be properly fed (and not overfed) because a new generation occurs about every four hours, and it is characteristic of all bacteria to develop unsuitable and even virulent strains depending on how they are fed."[13] When the diet contains too much sugar and too little fiber, the intestinal bacteria develop abnormal strains. This can lead to various diseases such as diverticulitis, colon infections, digestive and circulatory problems, diabetes, obesity, appendicitis, and gall bladder infections.*[14]

Professor Enderlein, former professor of zoology and microbiology at Berlin University, teaches that "all pathogenic germs are only phases in a developmental chain of one and the same congenital parasite existing in the blood of all human beings and other mammals."[15] If the balance between the mineral salts (alkali) and acids in the blood is disturbed by prolonged wrong nutrition resulting in acidosis, this parasite increases and brings about pathological changes. This is another variation on the theme that micro-organisms reflect and are symptomatic of the conditions of their environment, which in turn reflects the living habits of the host organism.

The pertussis vaccine, which has been implicated in so many cases of vaccine injury, is particularly difficult to produce precisely because the pertussis organism—Bordella pertussis—is so mutable! It has the ability to mutate unexpectedly and change its character. Even carefully selected strains perform differently when grown in different media, John Cameron of the University of Quebec tells us.[16]

Can the human mind induce mutations in bacteria? At St. Joseph's University in Philadelphia, 52 human volunteers not known to be psychically gifted, promoted the mutation of bacteria from one strain to another simply by "wishing." Conversely, they were able to inhibit the reverse mutation by the same mental intention.[17]

If thought, which is energy, can influence matter; then light, which is another form of energy, can also influence matter. All matter—atoms,

---

*Dr. Robinson tells of a year-long experiment in which five groups of baboons were fed different kinds of carbohydrates. The first four groups were fed refined carbohydrates— either glucose, fructose, sucrose (table sugar), or starch. The fifth group was fed natural foods such as bananas, yams, oranges, carrots, and bread. Only the animals in the first four groups showed demonstrable damage to the heart artery and a 35 percent rise in cholesterol. (See note 13 of this chapter.)

molecules, micro-organisms—gives off radiant energy which under certain conditions can be made visible. Royal Raymond Rife discovered that micro-organisms give off a monochromatic wave length of invisible ultra-violet light, and that a particular type of micro-organism disintegrates when subjected to a specific short wave frequency. Other frequencies would cause the micro-organism to illuminate or give off visible light, implying that these frequencies were vitalizing to the microorganism. Dr. Rife found he could save the lives of test animals that had been given lethal doses of pathogenic organisms by subjecting their bodies to the proper wave length of electrical energy, in this case, the oscillatory rate that would destroy the particular pathogen.[18] Are we moving toward the time when health care programs will include periodic exposure to specific life-enhancing radiation frequencies? We know that certain sounds and certain kinds of music have a therapeutic effect, while other sounds and other kinds of music have a disabling or debilitating effect.[19] And, of course, color therapy is an ancient art from which many have benefited.

"There is a surfeit of clinical information suggesting that we have literally become malnourished and sickened by the habitual diet of an outmoded view of the world, the classical Cartesian-Newtonian* description of the universe," writes Larry Dossey, M.D. He goes on to say that "this fragmented and alienated world view has directly contributed to fragmented and alienated life styles—with corresponding disease-ridden results."[20] The remedy, he says, is to incorporate a truer, more health-inducing picture of the world.

We know, for instance, that matter originates from and disappears into energy or force fields. "The world at bottom is a quantum energy world," physicist John Wheeler points out.[21] Yet we still think and act as though biochemical analysis were the final revelation. Most medical doctors and chemists, for example, have insisted that synthetic (manmade) food supplements are the same as natural food supplements (derived from food sources and processed in such a way as to retain enzymes and other nutrients) because their chemical formula is the same. Now we know that not only do the atoms in the molecules of the synthetic product rotate differently from the atoms of the natural one,** but the natural product has a more dynamic energy pattern than the synthetic.

---

*The world seen in terms of discrete objects and subject/object dualism.

**"The plane of a beam of polarized light is rotated by all natural substances either to the left (l-form) or to the right (d-form). Substances not occurring in nature may not cause rotation of the plane of polarization and these substances are said to be optically inactive (dl-form)." (Beatrice Trum Hunter, "Synthetic Vitamins," *Consumers' Research Magazine*, March 1974, p. 19.)

Two researchers, Drs. Justa Smith and Ehrenfried Pfeiffer, have demonstrated with a series of chromatograms—photographs that reproduce the energy patterns of an object (somewhat like Kirlian photography)—that natural substances have an energy pattern characterized by "radial lines and fluted edges, while the pattern of the synthetic product is almost entirely concentric and relatively dull looking."[22] Looking at these chromatograms, one begins to feel that natural is indeed beautiful.

The characteristic pattern of a natural substance, e.g., orange juice or grape juice, is destroyed by pasteurization and some preservatives. The living pattern is diminished or weakened by freezing and by other preservatives. In other words, as a method of food preservation, freezing is less destructive than heat, and some preservatives are more destructive than others. Even food grown in soil in which the compost had been sterilized showed fewer "live" elements than food grown in compost that was not heat treated. "There is a delicate and admirable balance of components in all the kingdoms of nature, Dr. Smith points out. And this balance is disturbed not only by refining out nutrients but by adding preservatives like BHA and BHT."[23]

What are the live elements that give the natural product its characteristic pattern and look of aliveness? They are enzymes and, as we learned earlier, they are destroyed by heat above 122 degrees Fahrenheit.

Over a hundred years ago, Bechamp discovered the difference between natural and synthetic substances. He found that chalk buried in limestone brought about fermentation whereas chemically "pure" chalk (calcium carbonate) made in his laboratory would not. What was in the natural chalk, buried for thousands of years in the ground, that did not exist in the chemically pure chalk? It was the microzymas, of course; their secretions—products of metabolism—are the enzymes that cause fermentation.

Fish or sea vegetation cannot live in synthetic sea water although it is chemically identical with the real thing; however, when just one ounce of real sea water is added to 20 gallons of the synthetic substitute, that "something" the chemists are unable to isolate or analyze changes the water so that fish and sea plants can live in it.[24] Is this living "something" the microzymas?

It is tempting to ask, "At what point does matter become energy?" Royal Raymond Rife discovered when he looked into his Universal Microscope that cells "are actually composed of smaller cells, themselves made up of even smaller cells, this process continuing with higher and higher magnification in a sixteen-step, stage-by-stage journey into the micro-beyond."[25] Bechamp stressed the almost invisible size as well as the "immeasurableness" of microzymas. Are they the elemental living principle?*

Generally, doctors using natural methods of healing have long advocated the use of natural substances in preference to their synthetic counterpart, saying in effect, that because these substances are biologically active they are more effectively utilized by the body. Medical literature contains numerous reports confirming this idea. One report, for instance, states that cases of scurvy failed to respond to synthetic vitamin C and that a cure was effected only when the patients were given a natural food substance containing vitamin C.[26]

Part of the aliveness of natural foods and food supplements is that they are wholistic; that is, they contain associated nutritional elements such as enzymes, co-enzymes, and trace minerals, as well as vitamins and minerals which assist in the process of assimilation. Many of these food elements have yet to be discovered.

A beautiful health care system would be holistic on many levels, focusing on parts only as they relate to and harmonize with a larger whole. It would see the body-mind as a purposive, dynamic energy field to be responded to, not a machine or an inert mass to be manipulated. A beautiful health care system would focus on the patient and his uniqueness, not on disease and herd remedies such as mass inoculations. And above all, it would be open-minded, aware that truth has many dwelling places and that our senses and our intellect apprehend only a fraction of the living universe.

THE "UGLY" SOLUTION

Whoever has the mind to fight has broken his connection with the universe.

TERRY DOBSON, QUOTING HIS AIKIDO TEACHER, "A SOFT ANSWER"

Disease Wars

We speak of "delivering a knockout punch to leukemia," "fighting multiple sclerosis," "battling muscular dystrophy", and "waging a war

---

*Thomas Edison apparently had an understanding of this principle when he wrote, "Take our own bodies. I believe they are composed of myriads and myriads of infinitesimally small individuals, each in itself a unit of life, and that these units work in squads—or swarms as I prefer to call them—and that these infinitesimally small units live forever. When we die these swarms of units, like a swarm of bees, so to speak, betake themselves elsewhere, and go on functioning in some other form or environment." (The Diary and Sundry Observations.)

against cancer." In fact, we not only fight disease, we fight litter, poverty, pornography, crime, mediocrity, and, yes, even fat. If we are confronted with a challenge—usually called a "problem"—we must "fight" it.

At the Center for Attitudinal Healing in California, children with "life-threatening" diseases draw pictures of "getting well." One picture shows "bad cells" lining up on one side and "good cells" lining up on the other. All cells are carrying guns. Another drawing shows two "bad cells" being attacked by a fighter plane driven by "good cells." In the bottom right hand corner is a tank labeled "good cells" which is also attacking the "bad cells." In another drawing, a circle with the label "angel" is sending lightening darts to a figure labeled "devil."[27]

For over a century we have used metaphors of fight, attack, and defend to describe our relationship with disease. The military mentality which creates these metaphors is also the mentality that designs weapons. A good weapon is supposed to destroy the enemy without harming the soldier who uses it. The problem is, it doesn't quite work that way. Aside from the more subtle level of psychic and quantum energies in which the universe reveals itself as a tissue of interconnections and reciprocal relationships, there is the gross, sensate level of reality in which the entrance of destructive energies at one level of an ecosystem reverberates on many levels of that system and even other systems as well. Simply stated, any remedy powerful enough to destroy "the other" destroys the host as well. The destruction of the host may be slower, the debilitating effects more subtle and long range, but the weapons approach to a challenge—whether on a microscopic scale involving cellular particles or on a macroscopic scale involving international relations—signifies the old consciousness of separation, materiality, and inanimateness.

"If there should be life on the moon, we must begin by fearing it. We must guard against it, lest we catch something," Lewis Thomas tells us after describing the elaborate, antiseptic ceremony through which the astronauts must pass on their return to earth in order to become members once again of the human community. "It is remarkable that we have all accepted this, without hooting, as though it simply conformed to a law of nature. It says something about our century, our attitude toward life, our obsession with disease and death, our human chauvinism." Further on, he points out that "most of the associations between the living things we know about are essentially cooperative ones, symbiotic in one degree or another." In discussing bacteria, he says that "they should provide nice models for the study of interactions between forms of life at all levels. They live by collaboration, accommodation, exchange, and barter."[28]

Back in 1903, Russian biologist, Peter Kropotkin, wrote a book called *Mutual Aid: A Factor of Evolution* in which he amassed almost as much evidence that animals cooperate as Darwin did that each is engaged in a selfish struggle for existence.[29] Are we reaping the final fruits of our predisposition to interpret events in combative, competitive terms in an armaments race that threatens to extinguish life on this planet?

"War is an old habit of thought, an old frame of mind, an old political technique, that must now pass as human sacrifice and human slavery have passed," writes Herman Wouk in his preface to *War and Remembrance*. Will we outgrow this habit, this old frame of mind before it is too late? As Buckminster Fuller has said, "We are in our final exams."

It is probably no accident that one of the major drug cartels, I. G. Farben (Germany), is also a major munitions manufacturer and a former designer and operator of the extermination camps used in Nazi Germany.[30] The weapons mentality wages wars on many levels.

The war game is, as many have observed, exceedingly profitable for the munitions industry, in this case, the pharmaceutical-medical industry. In 1981, for instance, vaccine distribution of eight major vaccines in the United States generated $300 million for the drug industry.[31]

Propaganda to keep enlistments up and money rolling in is part of the war machinery. The appeal to fear and the necessity for technological intervention and management of disease is illustrated in much of the literature distributed by state departments of health. "The hidden menace" and "killer and crippler" are some of the terms used to describe certain childhood infectious diseases from which children must be "protected" by immunizations. "Danger," "warning," "allowed to strike" are some of the scare terms used to intimidate parents into getting their children immunized. The more serious consequences as well as the frequency of the disease for which children are given immunizations are maximized if not grossly exaggerated, while the frequency of serious complications resulting from vaccinations is ignored or greatly minimized.

Superstitions, like old soldiers, never die. They simply change clothes and sit in the seats of respectability. Medical historian Henry E. Sigerist, M.D., points out:

> Primitive man found himself in a magical world, surrounded by a hostile nature whose every manifestation was invested with mysterious forces. In order to live unharmed, he had to use constant vigilance and had to observe a complicated system of rules and

rites that protected him from the evil forces which emanated from nature and his fellow men.[32]

Let's look at a folder distributed by the Virginia State Department of Health. In the middle section is a schedule which reads as follows:

2 months	DTP, TOPV
4 months	DTP, TOPV
6 months	DTP
15 months	Measles
	Rubella
	Mumps
18 months	DTP, TOPV
4 to 6 years	DTP, TOPV
14 to 16 years	Td

Does this look a bit like a reappearance of the "complicated system of rules and rites" primitive man lived by in order to protect himself from the evil forces which surrounded him? Have the miracle cures primitive man sought in the spells and potions of the witch doctor become the "miracle cures" of drugs and vaccines? The above schedule is only the beginning, of course. Biochemists and virologists are now looking for vaccines for AIDS, herpes, cancer, arthritis, and even leprosy. A new meningitis vaccine has recently been approved and recommended for every American child who has reached the age of two. It is a short step from recommendation to coercion as anyone familiar with the history of vaccination can attest. Once the paradigm is brought into—the idea of carriers and protection—the possibilities for exploitation and coercion are almost endless, and becoming a human pin cushion seems perfectly sensible.

Why are these unnatural approaches to health—vaccines and drugs—not beautiful compared to the more natural approaches we discussed earlier? Not only do unnatural (meaning dependent upon synthetic drugs and a complex technology) treatments ultimately complicate the disease process, but they escalate cost, dependency, and concentration of power outside of oneself. Perhaps, even more important, they promote a sense of alienation from one's own body and the natural world that sustains it. The body is not seen as an extension of one's consciousness and part of a larger continuum that includes all life, but as an isolated object that must fight for survival and defend itself against a hostile environment.

TABLE 3. TWO APPROACHES TO HEALTH CARE

THE "UGLY" SOLUTION	THE "BEAUTIFUL" SOLUTION
1. Atomized, fragmented.	1. Holistic—parts integrated and understood in relation to larger wholes.
2. Focuses on data and effects.	2. Focuses on principles and underlying causes.
3. Adversarial—promotes feelings of alienation.	3. Harmonious—promotes feelings of connection and relatedness.
4. Focuses on negative— engenders fear.	4. Focuses on positive— inspires.
5. Circuitous—skirts around the real problem.	5. Direct—goes to the core of the problem.
6. Obfuscating, complicating.	6. Clarifying.
7. Externalizes causality.	7. Internalizes causality.
8. Capricious, arbitrary.	8. Orderly, logical.
9. Superficial and simplistic.	9. Elegantly simple and multidimensional.
10. Addictive—creates dependency.	10. Empowering—supports autonomy and self-responsibility.
11. Wasteful—cost escalating.	11. Economical—cost effective.
12. Closed shop—authoritarian.	12. Open ended—egalitarian.
13. Short range.	13. Long range.
14. Side effects.*	14. Side benefits.

*A friend of mine, E. Dana Congdon, M.D., told a group of us that since he switched from using drugs in his practice to using herbs, he no longer worried about side effects in his patients, but could look forward to seeing side benefits.

The ugly solution is fragmented, superficial and short range. It looks for the immediate, the obvious, the quick fix. Because it focuses on the management of symptoms rather than the correction of causes, it lacks a unifying principle. Like the old pantheon of deities and devils, the ugly solution externalizes causality and promotes feelings of victimization and dependence on the expert. Geared to profits for the professional, it eschews the promotion of self-responsibility and independence.

As we move from a mass to an energy consciousness, from the

model of the body as a machine composed of discrete parts set on automatic, to a model of the body as an energy ecosystem directed by a consciousness, a monolithic, adversarial health care system will be increasingly hard to justify. How can we begin to transform a limited vision and ugly solutions into a larger vision suggesting more beautiful solutions?

"Nature is a part of us, as we are a part of it. We can recognize ourselves in the description we give it,"[33] physical chemist and Nobel laureate Ilya Prigogine points out. We need to recognize the combativeness within ourselves when we see the world as a mosaic of adversarial relationships. As author and educator, Noel McInnes said, "Complete emancipation of our latent powers is not possible as long as we are enthralled by the mentality of attack."[34] When we transform an adversarial consciousness—the consciousness of attack and defend—into a consciousness of connectedness, cooperation, and compassion, the beautiful solution will reveal itself.

NOTES

1. "Beauty, simplicity, harmony keys to physics, neuroscience, art and music," *Brain/Mind Bulletin*, Dec. 10, 1984, p. 2.
2. Ibid.
3. John Holt, *Instead of Education*, E. P. Dutton, Inc., New York, 1976, p. 91. John Holt is discussing a point made by Wertheimer in his book, *Productive Thinking*.
4. Paul Pietsch, "The Mind of a Microbe," *Science Digest*, Oct. 1983, pp. 69–71, 103. Also, "Wishing spurs genetic mutation in bacteria," *Brain/Mind Bulletin*, Sept. 10, 1984, p. 1.
5. William McGarey, M.D., "The Temple Beautiful," A.R.E. at Virginia Beach, Va., July 6, 1981.
6. Mary Coddington, *In Search of The Healing Energy*, Warner/Destiny Books, New York, 1978, p. 14.
7. Ibid. p. 98.
8. Ibid.
9. Bernard Jensen, D.C., N.D., *The Science and Practice of Iridology*, Bernard Jensen Products Publishing Division, Escondido, Calif., 1952, pp. 31–32.
10. Bernard Jensen, D.C., N.D., *You Can Master Disease*, Bernard Jensen Publishing Division, Solana Beach, Calif., 1952, p. 208.
11. Robert C. Olney, M.D., "Blocked Oxidation," (a reprint), *Cancer News Journal*, Vol. 8, no. 5, 1973.

12. Ibid.
13. Miles Robinson, M.D., "On Sugar and White Flour . . . the Dangerous Twins!" *Executive Health*, Vol. XI, No. 6. Referred to and quoted from in the article "Don't Eat Sugar!" Better Nutrition, April 1980, pp. 19, 38.
14. Ibid.
15. "Liver Damage as the Cause of Cancer and All Precanceroses," E. L. David, F.I.S.Ph. (Biological Researcher from England), *Cancer Control Journal*, Vol. 3, No. 1 & 2, 1975, p. 52.
16. Harris L. Coulter and Barbara Loe Fisher, *DPT: A Shot in the Dark*, Harcourt Brace Jovanovich, New York, 1985, p. 27.
17. "'Wishing' spurs genetic mutation in bacteria," *Brain/Mind Bulletin*, Sept. 10, 1984, p. 1.
18. Royal Lee, D.D.S., "The Rife Microscope or 'Facts and Their Fate,' " Reprint No. 47, The Lee Foundation for Nutritional Research, Milwaukee, Wisc. Also, Christopher Bird, "What has become of the Rife Microscope?" *New Age*, March 1976, pp. 41–47.
19. Steven Halpern and Louis Savary, *Sound Health: The Music and Sounds that Make Us Whole*, Harper and Row, San Francisco, 1985.
20. Larry Dossey, "Space, Time, and Medicine," *ReVision*, Fall, 1982, p. 57.
21. Ibid. p. 56.
22. Jane Kinderlehrer, "'Natural' is Beautiful—and Better!", *Prevention*, Jan. 1974, p. 97.
23. Ibid. p. 99.
24. "Natural vs. Synthetic: What is the Real Answer?" *Organic Consumer Report*, Feb. 27, 1962.
25. Christopher Bird, "What has become of the Rife Microscope?" *New Age Journal*, Mar. 1976, p. 41.
26. Beatrice Trum Hunter, "Synthetic Vitamins," *Consumers' Research Magazine*, March 1974, p. 18.
27. Center for Attitudinal Healing, *There is a Rainbow Behind Every Dark Cloud*, Celestial Arts Publishers, Millbrae, Calif., 1979.
28. Lewis Thomas, *The Lives of a Cell*, Bantam Books, New York, 1980, pp. 6–7.
29. Tom Bethell, "Burning Darwin to Save Marx," *Harpers*, Dec. 1978, p. 38.
30. Peter Barry Chowka, "Pushers in White: The Organized Drugging of America," *East/West Journal*, March 1979, p. 32.
31. Harris L. Coulter and Barbara Loe Fisher, *DPT: A Shot in the Dark*, Harcourt, Brace, Jovanovich, New York, 1985, p. 406.
32. Henry E. Sigerist, *Civilization and Disease*, Cornell University Press, Ithaca, N.Y., 1943, p. 131.

33. Quoted by Larry Dossey, M.D., in *Space, Time and Medicine*,
    Shambhala, Boulder, Colo., 1982, p. 82.
34. Noel McInnis, "Living Without Attack," *Green Light News*, May
    1984, p. 6.

PART III

■

FREE TO CHOOSE

A free society, if it is to remain free, cannot permit itself to be dominated by one strain of thought.

WILLIAM J. BAROODY, SR.

9

■

APPOINTMENT
WITH TYRANNY

*The condition of freedom in any state is always a
widespread and consistent skepticism of the canons upon
which power rests.*

HAROLD J. LASKI

"IT'S THE LAW"

On August 19, 1981, a social worker rang the doorbell at our residence
in Virginia and informed us that a member of our family, a young person
in excellent health, was required by law to submit to a medical procedure
which was not only fraught with risk, but was not even guaranteed to
be effective! The medical procedure was immunization, and the young
person was my 2 ½-year-old grandson, Isaac, who was living with us
at the time. Tanya, Isaac's mother and my daughter, was also living
with us. (She was separated from her husband.)

Since Tanya was at work, the social worker left a letter in a sealed
envelope for her. The letter told her to call and make an appointment
to see the social worker, Deborah Balak, within the next two days.

"The social worker was certainly pleasant and agreeable," I told

Tanya. "But she did say it was against the law not to have your child vaccinated. I told her it was not against the law because I had a copy of the Virginia law and it allowed two exemptions—medical and religious. I also told her there was an impressive body of medical opinion and empirical evidence indicating that this practice was harmful. I told her we had never had our children vaccinated. She said she didn't want to harass us but was merely doing her duty."

"So this is what happens when you tell the truth. I probably should never have taken him to the hospital!" Tanya replied. She was referring to the emergency hospital where she had taken Isaac a few days earlier (August 14) to see if he needed stitches. (He had fallen from the couch and had cut his head on the edge of the coffee table.) During the course of the examination, the nurse asked if he were "caught up with his shots." Tanya, being "oriented" on this issue, replied, "Ohhhhhhhh no!"

"This shouldn't take long, Tanya. Just give her a copy of the exemption form we used in California stating that immunizations are contrary to your beliefs," I told her.

On August 21 Tanya went to see the social worker and presented her with the signed vaccination exemption form I had used in California. Naively, I had assumed this was a national provision. Deborah told Tanya her stand was contrary to law and she would have to report it to the judge. She gave Tanya a copy of the law and Tanya said in parting, "This better not take much of my time!"

A few days later, Tanya received a summons to appear in court with Isaac on September 8, 1981.

When we read the summons we were shocked. It stated that the parents or guardian of William Isaac Turner "observe reasonable conditions of behavior pending final determination of custody to wit: to refrain from acts of commission or omission which tend to endanger the child's life, health or normal development." When Tanya read this, she had nightmares of someone taking her beautiful, adored Isaac away from her. I must confess I shared some of this nightmare myself, particularly when I remembered the Chad Green case.[1]

WE GO TO COURT

September 8: Tanya, Isaac, and I sat for two and a half hours on the hard benches of Room 201, District Courts Building, waiting for the name "Turner" to be called. I went along to help take care of Isaac and to give my daughter moral support. As it turned out, however, I did everything I had counseled my daughter not to do. I lost my cool.

We had brought along a folder full of medical statements indicating both the harmfulness and ineffectiveness (ineffective in terms of doing what it is supposed to do) of the practice of vaccination. Most of these statements were taken from material that appeared in Chapter 2 of this book. We also had a letter from our local medical doctor, Paul Monroe (not his real name). The letter stated that the child did not need routine vaccinations because of "possible dangers to his health" based on "national medical statements indicating the dangers of vaccinations." We also had another exemption form signed by Tanya which stated that vaccinations were contrary to her religious beliefs. We thought we were covered. We would present the letter and the evidence to the judge and that would be the end of it. How naive we were!

At 1:30 the name "Turner" was called and we went to another courtroom. Tanya sat on one side, Deborah Balak and a gentleman whose function we did not know sat on the other side, and Isaac and I sat in the audience section facing the judge. After the charges were read, Tanya opened her folder and presented the letter from Dr. Monroe to the judge. The judge waved it in the air and said, "Who is this Dr. Monroe? What does F.A.C.S. mean? This is no exemption letter." Approximately the next five or 10 minutes went something like this:

JUDGE:	We need a statement from a pediatrician. Where is the child's pediatrician?
ME:	We don't have one. This is an invasion of privacy.
TANYA:	There is a great deal of evidence that vaccinations are harmful.
ME:	Yes, Rutgers; U.C., California; Dr. Mendelsohn.
JUDGE:	Well, we'll see. I've had all my children vaccinated.
ME:	There is a religious exemption.
JUDGE:	(waving his arms) Ohhhh no!

A few exchanges with the social worker and Tanya, which I have forgotten, and then the judge said, "Well, you'll need to get a lawyer."

ME:	This better not cost anything. We're not paying a cent!

At this point the judge reprimanded me for being disorderly and ordered me to leave the court. Tanya told me to take Isaac with me, which I did. In his reprimand the judge said that this case was between the Commonwealth of Virginia and Mrs. Turner, not me. As I was walking out into the parking lot with Isaac, I thought, "This case is not between the state of Virginia and Tanya; it is between freedom and tyranny."

After the court hearing was adjourned, Tanya talked in the hall with Deborah Balak and the gentleman who was with her in the courtroom. Later we discovered he was Michael Soberick, the prosecuting attorney. When Tanya came to the parking lot she told me, "That man with Deborah wanted to see the letter from Dr. Monroe. He told me to get him to rewrite the letter to read more like the law and he would be satisfied and drop the case. But I don't want to bother Dr. Monroe anymore. I told them I could take the religious exemption. The man asked me what my religion was, and I told him, 'My own private religion.' He sort of snickered when I said that." Tanya also told me that he seemed to want to get the whole thing over with and that it was Deborah who was pressing the issue.

Tanya also told me the judge appointed a lawyer for Isaac and asked her how much she made so he could suggest a lawyer for her. She declined to divulge her salary because she felt it was none of the court's business. (She was working as a computer programmer.) The judge, therefore, did not suggest a lawyer.

When Tanya told me this, I was outraged. So this was going to cost money as well as more time and energy! We had broken no law that I knew of and yet Tanya was being charged with the expense not only of a defense attorney for herself but very possibly for the state-appointed attorney for her child. (The summons stated on the reverse side that the parents could be charged with the cost of the legal services for their child.)

Perhaps the real irony of the whole affair was that it would be hard to find a child more loved and carefully reared than Isaac. Tanya stayed home form work for over two years to nurse him, and he was fed only fresh, whole, "natural" foods and food supplements.

That night I had insomnia. The spectre of possible large legal fees and more time and energy down the drain kept me awake. (Our financial resources could best be described as modest.) My daughter told me the next morning that she also slept poorly. To people uninitiated in the ways of the mindless machinery of the state legal system, the experience of confronting its police powers can be frightening. (When I use the term "mindless" I mean mind plugged into automatic and thereby disconnected from its perceptive and reflective powers.)

FIRST AID ARRIVES

The next day I called the National Health Federation in Monrovia, California. This is an organization whose purpose is to promote freedom of choice in health matters. When I explained our problem, the secretary connected me to Clinton Miller, the Federation's Legislative Advocate. We discussed both the medical and religious exemptions that were allowed in the state of Virginia, and it became apparent that taking the religious exemption was by far the easier and less expensive way to go. Clinton had a letter written to Deborah and a statement for us to sign which said that "the administration of immunizing agents conflicts with their religious tenets and practices." He would have sent a letter to the judge had we known his name.

Talking with Clinton was very therapeutic. The tension of being alone and not knowing drained out of me. Tanya had much the same experience when I relayed the information to her that evening.

Three days later Clinton's letter arrived. We—both parents and maternal grandparents—signed the statement. Monday morning, September 14, Tanya delivered to the social worker the envelope containing the letter, the signed statement, and the religious exemption form which she had not had a chance to present to the judge the week before.

On September 21 Deborah called Tanya at work to make an appointment to discuss the letter Tanya had given her. Two days later Tanya and Alan (her husband) visited Deborah in her office. She said she felt the letter misrepresented her because Tanya had merely said that vaccination was against her beliefs, not religious beliefs. She inquired about Tanya's religious beliefs. Tanya said that the specific religious tenet that the practice of vaccination violated was her belief that the body was the temple of God and the use of immunizing agents polluted the body. In other words, her religious practices included not using immunizing agents. Deborah was not sufficiently impressed to call the whole thing off and said to Alan, "You know, of course, it's important to have the child protected." Tanya told me she seemed genuinely concerned about the welfare of the child.

Lawyers and Churches

On September 25 Tanya called Clinton Miller to tell him that the letter did not deter Ms. Balak from pursuing legal action against her and to ask him what course of action he would now recommend. He recommended we engage Gerald Norton (not his real name) as our attorney. Tanya then asked if there were any possibility of our losing the case. Clinton implied it was not inconceivable because we were up against a tyranny. Tanya replied she would leave the state before she would have Isaac vaccinated. Clinton mentioned the possibility of raising funds for the defense.

Tanya went to see Gerald Norton about taking the case. He said he couldn't because he was going to Europe, and besides he would charge too much. (He said this after questioning her as to her financial status.) He recommended that she consult Joseph Connelly (not his real name), another lawyer, saying that the case was interesting and could easily go to the supreme court.

When Tanya went to see Joe Connelly, he read my account of the proceedings thus far and looked over the pertinent documents. Then he asked Tanya about her financial resources. When he found that these were inadequate, he recommended that she join the Christian Science Church "to take care of the immediate situation" (translate "get the law off your back"). When Tanya remonstrated that she would like to fight this very unjust law—which violates the very essence and spirit of democracy—and "open a few eyes," Joe said that the most feasible way for her in her financial position to go about doing this would be to write legislators and contact key people after the trial.

Earlier, Joe Connelly had contacted the city attorney who was sitting with Deborah Balak at the initial hearing. The attorney said that being a member of the Christian Science Church would satisfy the law. He also said that getting the doctor to write a letter stating that the child had some specific physical condition for which inoculations were contraindicated would satisfy the law. Obviously we couldn't ask a doctor to lie because Isaac is a healthy child.

The disappointing aspect of this experience for Tanya was that no one seemed really interested in her case, not even the principle of the thing which is our real bone of contention. (The principle being, of course, the right of freedom of choice in personal health care matters.) The lawyers were only interested in somehow satisfying the letter of the law and obtaining money for their services. She finally learned that hiring lawyers and going to court—especially for the purpose of defending a principle—is a rich man's game.

She told us she planned to go to the Christian Science Church and get an application for membership.

That Sunday, October 4, Tanya came home early from an out-of-town trip in order to go to the Christian Science Church. She had been to the Christian Science Reading Room earlier in the week and had gotten some literature and read it. The ideas, for the most part, were congenial and so she went to the church. She came home happy with what she found, saying the people were warm and friendly. She got an application for membership.

The next day I called the American Civil Liberties Union in Richmond, Virginia to see if they would take a case like ours. The girl answering the phone told me that they were so far behind in litigation that they could take no new cases; and before they could take our case, it would have to be reviewed by a board. She gave me the impression that it was not beyond the realm of possibility for them to take a case such as ours, the only criterion being whether a civil liberty was being violated.

On Wednesday, October 7, Clinton Miller called. In essence he said that he felt it was wrong for anyone to join a church under coercion and that the advice the lawyer gave Tanya is referred to in legal parlance as "expeditious" advice. In other words, if you don't have the money to afford a lawyer just do something to get yourself off the hook. I gave him Joe Connelly's phone number, and he said he was going to write some letters and make some phone calls. He told us to call him at his home on Saturday if we hadn't heard from him. We decided, however, that we would simply go to court and Tanya would say in effect, "I can't afford a lawyer. These are my religious tenets and practices and this right is protected by the constitution. Religion is a very private and personal thing not to be defined or limited by the state." Also, Clinton said that it was not beyond the realm of possibility that the Christian Science Church would not accept her and then where would she be. Certainly, his own church would turn down an application if the person applying appeared motivated by any other reason than deeply felt commitment to the tenets of the church.

When Tanya got home she called Clinton and told him of her "conversion" to the Christian Science Church. She said that the ideas of the church were congenial for the most part and that joining this church might solve other problems for her such as providing a Sunday school for Isaac. Clinton questioned the sincerity of her convictions, but when he realized that she seemed content with this solution, he said he would drop the case. He told her to call Michael Soberick, the prosecuting attorney, and maybe they would drop the hearing.

Tanya called Michael Soberick the next day and told him she had applied for membership in the Christian Science Church to satisfy the law. He said that in that event the case would be continued for six months at which time it would be reviewed to be sure she was still a member of the church in good standing. He asked for the name of a person from the church who knew her and knew of her intentions to join. He also said they would require verification of her attendance.

Tanya then called me and was indignant. She said, "Well, I'm back to square one." The realization that she was going to be monitored and her sincerity checked, shattered her former enthusiasm; she recognized she had been motivated by expediency. I told her to call Clinton Miller and get his advice. She did and he laughed at her sudden "unconversion." They discussed writing a press release and getting publicity. He also mentioned Kirpatrick Dilling, the National Health Federation's lawyer in Chicago, and implied that the case would not be at all difficult for him to win. However, the concern was more with raising the level of public awareness than just winning the case. He told Tanya to have me write a press release and to call back later that evening with the article. He gave her the first sentence.

The next day Clinton called and we worked over the press release. I also talked with Jo Ludwig about starting an N.H.F. chapter here. They said they would send a packet of materials I would need to start a chapter.

Two days before the second court hearing (October 11), I awoke at 2 A.M. I went downstairs, took a pencil and several pieces of scratch paper, and wrote Tanya's defense speech. Later that morning I typed it up; Paul, my husband and Tanya's father, edited it, and Tanya made a few changes. She practiced the speech in front of us. We made a few suggestions.

IN COURT AGAIN

October 13: Second Hearing. Tanya, Alan, Isaac, Paul, and Ingri (Tanya's younger sister) attended the hearing. I didn't go into the courtroom because I was too angry, embarrassed, and frustrated. Angry, because to me this whole business was such an obvious violation of civil liberties and these people couldn't see it. Embarrassed, because I had misbehaved in a court of law. Frustrated, because I felt like an anthropologist who had stumbled into a tribe of primitives and found herself forced to give homage to their taboos and fetishes. Yes, my prejudices were surfacing.

We were better prepared for this hearing than we were for the first one. Not only did Tanya bring the speech we had prepared, but she brought additional medical evidence as well. We also knew the name of the judge (Frederick Aucamp) and the identity of the prosecuting attorney, Michael Soberick.

After the hearing, Tanya, Alan, Paul, and Ingri told me what happened in the courtroom. Like the Japanese film, "Rashomon," each had a different version of the drama. Alan thought Tanya's inability to handle the rebuttal and cross examination disastrous; Paul thought everything worked out beautifully; and Ingri, although critical of Tanya's delivery, was generally pleased at the way things went. Tanya herself told a reporter, "I was really happy with the judge. He listened to all my arguments." This is part of the speech she read to the court:

Your Honor, Judge Aucamp, Assistant City Attorney, Mr. Soberick and Ms. Balak from the Virginia Beach Department of Social Services. If it pleases your Honor I would like approximately seven minutes of your time to state my case.

I, Tanya Turner, am appearing *pro se* before this court today. I am appearing in my own defense because I cannot afford the services of a lawyer. The state has appointed an attorney, Mr. Alan Rosenblatt, for my son, Isaac. Because I cannot afford his services either, I do not accept the services of Mr. Rosenblatt.

I am appearing in this court today because I am charged with failure to have my two-year-old son, Isaac, vaccinated. I believe this charge comes under the category of medical neglect. Since I deliberately chose not to have my son vaccinated, this is not a case of neglect but of educated choice. I chose not to have my son vaccinated for both medical and religious reasons. The state law of Virginia allows both these exemptions. I tried to satisfy the medical exemption by presenting to you, at the first hearing on September 8, 1981, a letter from our doctor, Paul Monroe, a general surgeon. You would not accept this letter. I would have attempted to satisfy the religious exemption at that time but was prevented from doing so.

. . . As an American citizen whose right to worship according to the dictates of his own conscience is protected by the Constitution of the United States, I object to the surveillance procedures Mr. Soberick has suggested. I refuse to be coerced into a particular form of worship.

Virginia State law says *nothing* about *organized* religion in the "religious tenets or practices" allowed in the first exemption. The notion that this exemption applies only to members of an organized religion is only an interpretation of some lawyers. This *interpretation* violates the First Amendment of the Constitution of the United States which I will read in part.

"Congress shall make no law respecting an establishment of religion, or prohibiting the free exercise thereof. . . ."

The state may not define what a religion is and is not. A religious tenet or practice is not limited to a tenet or practice of an *organized* religion. Religion is a personal and private matter and includes any sincerely held belief.

While I will continue to investigate the Christian Science

Church, I will base my defense at this time on my *own personal* religious tenets and practices. I believe that the body is the temple of God. This is a religious tenet, found in the Bible, First Corinthians, Chapter 6, Verse 19.

I, myself, have never been vaccinated. I do not believe in the injection of foreign and, therefore, toxic substances into the human body. My religious practices, therefore, include not using immunizing agents.

I have another religious tenet that is the very bedrock upon which this country was founded. I believe in freedom of choice. I believe the right of the individual to decide for himself how he will conduct the affairs of his life is sacred and inalienable as long as he injures no one else. If a person does not have the right to choose what shall be done to his own body and how he shall rear his own children, what right does he have?

Thank you, your Honor.

The judge listened courteously and asked for any witnesses. Ingri described how sick she became and how her hair fell out after a smallpox and cholera vaccination in India. After consulting Black's legal dictionary for the definition of religion, Judge Aucamp said that Tanya's objection to vaccination was really philosophical rather than religious and therefore didn't come under the protection of the First Amendment. He said in effect, "At the next hearing then, you'll have to present medical evidence that vaccinations are harmful or I'll have no other choice but to order shots for the child unless you appeal." He instructed Tanya to take the necessary medical evidence to the prosecuting attorney two weeks before the third hearing.

PUBLICITY AND NEW CONTACTS

On October 14, Tanya and Isaac's picture appeared in the *Virginian-Pilot* with an accompanying article entitled, "Woman challenges required vaccinations." "I refuse to be coerced into a particular kind of worship," she told the reporter after telling him how the city attorney's office had advised her that her membership in the Christian Science Church would be monitored over a period of months.

A number of people called expressing concern and sympathy. Several of them—including a local nurse and a chiropractor—gave us some valuable information which we included in our exhibit. We were also urged by several people to get a lawyer.

I wrote to Thomas Finn, head of the Freedom of Choice Law Center in Georgia, in reference to his article in the *Vegetarian Times*, "How to Avoid Compulsory Immunizations." I asked a question that the article raised and enclosed a newspaper article about our case.

A few days later Tom Finn called and offered to represent us without charge if we would pay his travel expenses to and from Virginia Beach and his lodgings. He pointed out several possible pitfalls with the way we were proceeding and seemed very concerned that we not jeopardize the freedom of choice health movement by losing our case. I assured him we would not lose and would call him back after discussing this matter with the rest of the family and Clinton Miller.

After consulting with the family and Clinton, we agreed to have Tom Finn represent us. This choice also required a Virginia lawyer because Tom is not licensed in the state of Virginia. Tanya was relieved because she had been uneasy about appearing pro se in court again.

On October 30, about two and a half weeks before the court hearing, Paul and I delivered to Michael Soberick's office almost 90 pages of scientific evidence and medical opinions attesting to the harmful effects of vaccination. After I sent Tom Finn the pertinent papers and my account of the case as well as a copy of the exhibit we sent to the prosecuting attorney, Tom phoned the prosecuting attorney and told him to give the exhibit to the judge.

On November 17, Isaac's birthday and the evening before the court hearing, we picked Tom up at the airport. Because we didn't know what he looked like, Isaac carried a sign reading "Welcome Tom Finn." Between Tom's briefcase and our sign, recognition was easy. Tom was friendly and congenial, and we enjoyed our visit with him.

COURT AND VERDICT

At 1:00 P.M. on November 18 we were in court. Outside the courthouse Tanya was interviewed by TV reporters; inside the courthouse she was interviewed by newspaper reporters. After about 15 or 20 minutes we all filed into the courtroom, newspaper and TV reporters filling the second row and family and friends the third row. A sandy-haired, bespectacled man, whom I later found out was an official of the health department, sat in the second row.

Judge Aucamp immediately asked for the doctor's letter. Tom gave it to him, and the judge suggested we try to get it reworded to comply with the law. Tom said he would call Dr. Monroe to get him to reword the letter. Because Wednesday is Dr. Monroe's day off, Tom called him at his home. When Dr. Monroe said he would rewrite the letter, the health officer took the phone and read him the "riot act." He told Dr. Monroe that people would now get the idea that all they had to do was go to him and they wouldn't have to be vaccinated. The prosecuting attorney made the same objection when Tom told the court we were getting the letter from the doctor rewritten as requested. Dr. Monroe told the health officer that shots would be detrimental in this case because the family was so opposed to them. (I wasn't present at this scene since it took place "offstage." Tom told us this later, saying that Dr. Monroe was really a "strong man.")

Judge Aucamp made a motion to adjourn the court and reconvene when we could present the letter from the doctor. After several suggestions we finally agreed to meet the next day. Tom asked if it were necessary for him to be there and the judge said no. All that was necessary was for the letter to be reworded and turned in.

A couple of unusual elements in this scenario are worth comment. The first was that the letter did not have to state a negative physical condition for which vaccinations would be contraindicated. Tom pointed out that the law did not specify that the condition had to be negative. (Our exhibit presented evidence that vaccinations could be harmful to *any* child.)

The second was that after setting a date for readjournment and before dismissing the court, the judge made the statement that he didn't want to get into the medical aspects of this case because that would be "opening a can of worms." I couldn't help translate this rather revealing statement as, "I have seen the evidence and found that it does exist—vaccinations are harmful—but I'm stuck with a law I have to uphold and constituents I don't want to antagonize so let's all get off the hook as gracefully as possible."

November 19: The Day of the Chestnuts. Second part of the third hearing: Michael Soberick turned in a spirited performance. Once again he objected to the "hearsay evidence" of the letter which the judge had said the day before was precisely what the law called for. He wanted to cross examine the doctor. He objected to the "contradiction" of the two letters (really the second was simply more specific than the first). And finally, he repeated again the old chestnut, "Society has rights." He put Tanya on the witness stand and quibbled about the difference between "status" and "condition" and objected again that there was no health problem with the child for which shots would be contraindicated. Tanya replied that the condition which the law referred to could be positive or negative, the law didn't specify.

Before the final ruling more chestnuts fell:

MICHAEL:	Society has rights.
JUDGE:	The individual has rights, too.
MICHAEL:	The child should be protected.
JUDGE:	That's the responsibility of the parents.

When Michael made the statement that failure to vaccinate Isaac threatened public health, I wondered if he had read any of the material we turned in to him. When the judge finally ruled in our favor, he turned to Mike and said, "Well, Mike, I know you feel like you've been railroaded." The judge also said that the responsibility to prevent similar exemptions rests with the legislature, not him. "Hmmmmmmmm," I thought, "so the name of this game is *Win, Don't Rock the Boat*, and *Pass the Buck*."

After the hearing I went up to the judge and thanked him for his decision and apologized for my behavior at the first hearing.

FALLOUT

The next morning when we tuned in to the 8:00 A.M. news broadcast, the first news we heard was:

> Three-year-old Isaac Turner won a victory in the Virginia Beach courts yesterday. The mother maintained that the risks involved with vaccination do not warrant vaccinating a healthy child.

When we opened the front page of the local news section of the *Virginian-Pilot* we read the headline: "JUDGE EXEMPTS CHILD FROM INOCULATIONS." In the article Judge Aucamp was quoted as saying, "The risks of the shots outweigh the benefits." The article went on to say that a spokeswoman for the health department said that studies by the Federal Center for Disease Control show there are greater risks in failing to vaccinate children. She said that one-half of one percent of the children eligible for vaccinations are granted exemptions on medical or religious grounds each year, and that about 65,000 children were vaccinated in Virginia last year.

When I read these figures, I couldn't help being appalled. How can a nation of sheep be a free people? Apparently no one questions the wisdom of a theory which says in effect that the best way to build health—and disease prevention subsumes under health—is to poison the body.* And even worse, apparently no one questions the studies

*Vaccines are poisons by definition.

and pronouncements of a monolith, particularly a monolith with such
an obvious vested interest in perpetrating a particular point of view. I
was reminded of what Alvin Toffler said: "We need to begin thinking
like the same revolutionaries who made the American form of government in the first place."[2]

The afternoon paper, the *Ledger Star*, printed an article with the
suggestive title, "Doctor's note saves boy from vaccination."

Three days later (November 23), the *Virginian-Pilot* published a
letter to the editor written by Dr. Thomas Rubio, Professor of Pediatrics, Eastern Virginia Medical School, entitled "Children haven't a
'right' to disease," saying that the judge's ruling "disregarded the rights
of the child to be protected against serious illnesses." He took exception
to the judge's statement that "the risk of the shots outweigh the benefits"
by referring to "the extensive experience with vaccinations in this country" and the "well documented" studies of the U.S. Public Health
Service and the "recommendations of the American Academy of Pediatrics." He also warned of dire consequences of failure to comply
with the required immunization program.

On November 27 an editorial appeared in the *Virginian-Pilot* called
"Immunize immunizations," which objected to both the decision of the
judge and the letter of the doctor which exempted Isaac from vaccination. The arguments were typical: The recitation of statistics which
show a decline in the number of infectious diseases and the attribution
of this decline primarily to the practice of vaccination. The editor warned
of epidemics to come if the practice of compulsory mass immunizations
is not strictly adhered to: "Whenever an epidemic of childhood disease
occurs, the outbreak is nearly always traceable to a falloff in inoculations." The editorial concluded by saying, "If the General Assembly
values the health gains from mass immunizations, it will inoculate the
system against subversion by a physician's say-so."

On December 6 the *Virginian-Pilot* published my rebuttal under
the title, "Vaccination is a political disease." Even though my letter
was considerably shortened, the editor managed to extract the salient
points which were: (1) the decline in infectious diseases was not due to
vaccination; (2) the harmful effects of vaccination are not negligible nor
do they affect just a minuscule percentage of the population; and (3)
advocates of compulsory immunization are, in fact, "advocating taking
away one of our basic freedoms—the freedom of choice referred to in
the Declaration of Independence as the right to 'life, liberty and the
pursuit of happiness.'" My letter continued, "you advocate imposing
your medical beliefs—and they are beliefs—on others in violation of
the Constitution."

On the 10th of December Tanya received a letter from her Virginia lawyer, Hank Sadler. He informed her that Michael Soberick, the prosecuting attorney, was appealing the ruling of the judge. When Tanya first showed me the letter, my reaction was visceral: "How could he," I thought. "Did he read any of the material we gave him? . . . Maybe he's under pressure from the health department . . . or is it pressure from the ego?" The real point of the exhibit, as I saw it, was not so much to show how harmful vaccinations are but what a wide latitude of disagreement there is among doctors—the "experts"—themselves. Some refuse to give this shot or that shot, and some give only one shot at one time and not at another, and some, in agreement with us, say "no thanks" to the whole business. Gray areas like this are hardly places where the police powers of the state belong.

Shortly after we received this letter I wrote to Clinton Miller telling him we had already spent over $800 on this case and simply couldn't afford to spend any more. The National Health Federation sent out a letter to raise funds for Tanya's legal expenses. Included in the letter was a reproduction of the newspaper article with Tanya and Isaac's picture, a press release written by Clinton Miller and me, and an eloquent letter written by Dr. Mendelsohn.

A few weeks after the letter went out, we began receiving calls from sympathetic and interested people from all parts of the country. Some of them sent valuable literature which I have included in the second chapter of this book. One woman from Michigan told me we should be working with our legislators to get the law changed. Some wanted to send money, and I told them to send it to the NHF Legal Fund for Tanya.

Among the many letters and phone calls that came in during the next few months, a particularly heart-rending letter told of "a dear friend" whose beautiful, healthy six-year-old son, who had never been ill, "died a hideous death" after vaccination. Subsequent letters described the mother as being adamantly opposed to vaccinations. She had let herself be pressured into submitting to the vaccination because otherwise her son would not have been admitted to school in New York. Shortly after the vaccination the child went to sleep and slept all afternoon. Each day thereafter he "became more and more listless until excruciating pains and high fever forced his admittance to the local hospital. After numerous operations and unbelievable suffering for seven months the child died a hideous death." The writer of the letter went on to say that the mother "did not sue the doctor as he was, by New York state law, required to vaccinate the child before he would be permitted to enter school."

For the first time in my life I could fully identify with people all over the world who are struggling for freedom and with the founders of our country who dedicated their lives to create a constitution that would guarantee liberty for its citizens. Somehow I realized on a deeper level that the central theme of human history was indeed freedom, as Lord Acton* had said, and that life without it wasn't worth living.

NOTES

1. See "A Matter of Life, Death, and Freedom," Peter Barry Chowka, *New Age*, Jan. and Feb. 1980.
2. From a talk by Alvin Toffler, reported in the University of Utah *Review*, Nov. 1975.

---

*Lord Acton was an eminent Cambridge historian who began in 1880 a series of books in which he planned to expound human freedom as history's central theme. He is the author of the famous saying: "Power corrupts and absolute power corrupts absolutely."

10

■

"LET
MY PEOPLE GO"

When Israel was in Egypt land,
Let my people go.
Oppressed so hard, they could not stand,
Let my people go.

"GO DOWN, MOSES," NEGRO SPIRITUAL

"Let my people go." I could still hear our high school glee club singing those lines. "Go down, Moses . . . Tell old pharaoh/To let my people go." Yes, freedom is the central theme of human history.

THE MEDICAL PHARAOH

What happened to the participants in our drama? Dr. Monroe almost lost his license. The Virginia Beach Medical Society cited him for unethical conduct for the exemption letter he wrote for us. "Personal choice means absolutely nothing to these people," he told me. "They want complete control over you."

To Dr. Monroe it was unethical to force a medical treatment—and particularly a risky medical treatment—upon an unwilling patient. To

147

the Virginia Beach Medical Society it was unethical to break rank—to
go outside one's specialty and go against the party line.

Tanya and Isaac fared better than Dr. Monroe. Through a simple
legal maneuver Tom Finn got Mike Soberick to call off the appeal. We
were free . . . for the time being.

Among the many phone calls I received—mostly from people wanting more information about vaccinations and how to avoid them—a
particularly interesting and helpful one came from a woman in Wisconsin. She said that she and her family wanted to move to Virginia
(her husband had an excellent job offer) but would not consider it if
they were going to be hassled about immunizations as we were. She
described the struggle they had in Wisconsin getting the exemption
based upon personal conviction reinstated. The exemption had been
part of the law once—the result of the hard work of many people—
and suddenly they discovered it wasn't there anymore. She said that a
legislator told her the pressure was from the federal level. I said, "Of
course. In 1962 there was a compulsory immunization bill before Congress that would have exempted no one, but it was defeated because
of the efforts of such groups as the Christian Scientists, the National
Health Federation, the Natural Hygienists, and others." "Yes," she
said, "the legislator here told me that they are now going about it by
getting just a few states at a time."

Later she sent me a tape of a doctor speaking out against immunizations at a Natural Hygiene Convention, part of which I used in
writing Chapter 2 of this book. She also sent me some literature and a
remarkable book, *The Hazards of Immunization*, by Sir Graham S.
Wilson, M.D., LL.D., F.R.C.P., D.P.H., published by the University
of London (1967), which chronicles complications and fatalities from
the use of serums and vaccines. The accounts are relayed simply and
dryly, most of the mishaps being attributed to such things as bacterial
contamination or faulty preparation. Opening the book at random, we
read on page 88: "Olin and Lithander (1948) describe an incident in
which three children injected intramuscularly at the same time with
convalescent measles serum prepared at a hospital laboratory became
ill within 6 to 8 hours. They suffered from high fever, vomiting, and
diarrhea, followed by somnolence, agitation and cyanosis. Two of them
died 14 and 18 hours after the injection." Further down the page we
read: "In this incident, which occurred in India in October 1902, 19
persons injected with plague vaccine contracted tetanus 5–6 days later
and all died within 7–10 days of their injection." Similar incidents are
recounted for 290 pages and reinforced by 20 pages of references.

Perhaps the most depressing feature of this book is not so much the bloodless numbers, statistics, and recitations of cripplings and fatalities, but the discouraging realization that man learns very slowly; his ability to penetrate the multiple layers of data and phenomena and arrive at a clearing where principles reveal themselves is apparently very limited at this time. Dr. Wilson makes it clear that he is no anti-vaccinationist, saying that even though "all forms of active and passive immunization are potentially dangerous is no condemnation of their use" (p. 6).

A NEW BEGINNING

It was now time to contact legislators and formally open an area chapter of the National Health Federation. On January 4, 1982, I mailed letters to the five House of Delegates and the three state senators of our district requesting that Section D of Article 3, Chapter 2 of the Code of Virginia (the compulsory immunization law) be amended to include an exemption based upon personal beliefs. I cited a number of other states that had this exemption as well as the unconstitutionality of the present law. Three delegates replied saying they would investigate the matter, and our senator from this area, Joe Canada, said he would send my letter to Legislative services to have a bill drafted.

On May 13, 1982, the Tidewater Chapter of the National Health Federation had its first meeting. Our first project was getting a petition signed which requested that the Compulsory Immunization Laws of Virginia be amended to provide for an exemption based upon personal conviction. The petition mentioned that there were 19 states that already had this exemption. An accompanying sheet listed, with references, some of the diseases and disabilities that have been linked to immunizations and pointed out that there are natural and harmless ways of preventing and treating so-called dread diseases for which vaccines are given.

By the third meeting it became apparent that we weren't getting enough signatures, so I handed out samples of a form letter to be sent to state legislators in September. The letter was checked by the group.

A couple of interesting confrontations occurred in connection with our petition-signing activities. Several people told stories of an occasional person who was hostile and indignant when confronted with the petition. One person, who is a member of a church which is health and nutrition conscious, told how her fellow church members shied away from her when she approached them with the petition, saying in effect that their pediatricians knew best.

Another incident occurred with regard to getting publicity for our meetings. The first time I submitted an announcement of our meeting to *The Beacon*, a section of our leading local newspaper, for inclusion in their "Community in Action" section the editors deleted the phrase "freedom of choice in health matters." The second time I submitted the notice of our meeting, I included the above phrase plus "Speaker and discussion: Compulsory Immunization." This notice never appeared in the paper. When I inquired as to why our notice was not published, I was informed by the girl in charge that it had been omitted at the downtown offices, probably for reasons of space, and that *The Beacon* does not guarantee publication of all notices anyway. When I remonstrated that several notices much longer than mine were printed, she replied that it is easier to delete a whole notice than to delete part of a longer one.

The third time I submitted the notice of our meeting it was printed, but both the phrase "freedom of choice in health matters" (which explains what the Health Federation is all about) and the name and subject of the speaker were omitted. (The speaker was speaking on "Alternative Cancer Therapies." She had been cured of terminal cancer by using a combination of the laetrile and Gerson therapies and her story had been printed by both the *Virginian-Pilot* and *Ledger-Star*.)

I decided it was time to write the editor. When we remember that Virginia is a state that is proud of its colonial heritage, of the monuments and relics associated with the founding of our country—which was founded upon the ideals of freedom and brotherhood—the story I am telling seems particularly ironic. *The Beacon* frequently publishes stories featuring the history and current use of these historical relics. In fact, the edition in which our truncated notice appeared featured a story on a historical park here. So after describing our problem with the "Community in Action" section of *The Beacon*, I said to the editor:

> "Could it be that freedom is a dirty word when used in the "wrong" context? Is it a noble, inspiring and beautiful word when associated with historical names, places and objects; but does it become obscene, irrelevant and cumbersome when applied to current events that threaten the power and prerogative of one of the tribal gods?
>
> "The founders of our country established a system of checks and balances to ensure equitable treatment of people and issues. They knew that unless they established checks on power and prerogative these easily become abusive. Where are the checks and balances in the area of the healing arts? Only one school of healing—medicine—is recognized in a court of law and only their par-

ticular point of view is endorsed and disseminated by the media. Stories are legion of doctors—medical or otherwise—who either break with that point of view or never bought it in the first place and who are remarkably successful in "curing" people of all manner of maladies, including "incurable" ones. Their reward: ostracism, persecution and, in many cases, confiscation of materials and loss of license. This abuse of power, because it is unchallenged by a system of checks and balances, is precisely what the National Health Federation was organized to counteract. Does *The Beacon* align itself with this abuse of power?

About a week later I received a phone call. No, it was not from the editor but from the girl who takes the notices. "The problem is with 'freedom of choice in health matters'," she said. "You have freedom of choice. You can choose the doctor and the hospital you want." "But you can't choose the kind of therapy or even the kind of doctor you want," I said. "What if I wanted to go to a naturopath or a homeopath? The former aren't even licensed in this state and the latter aren't even represented in this area, as far as I know. Also, what if I had cancer and decided I wanted laetrile or some other metabolic therapy? At best I would have a very difficult time getting it." I also pointed out that freedom to choose includes the right to treat and prevent illness in different ways, the compulsory immunization law being an obvious violation of this principle. "So it's a right to pursue a different philosophy of health. Your objections are philosophical," she said. "You might put it that way," I replied.

We had no more trouble getting notices of our meetings in *The Beacon*.

POLITICS

We sent form letters to Virginia legislators asking them to introduce legislation to amend the compulsory vaccination law to allow for an exemption based upon personal belief. The letter quoted statements from Dr. J. Anthony Morris, former chief vaccine control officer of the FDA, that "there is a great deal of evidence to prove that immunization of children does more harm than good" and that "there is no rationale for forcing immunization." We also included the famous statement on vaccination by Clarence Darrow: "If vaccination does what its advocates claim for it, the person who is vaccinated ought to be safe no matter whether anybody else is vaccinated or not." We pointed out that 19 states already have a personal exemption and concluded by saying that "the practice of vaccination is controversial and is hardly an area where the police powers of the state belong."

Most legislators didn't reply. Of the three that did, one said he agreed and would support our position, but he was up for reelection and lost. One said he would study the matter, and another said he "had occasion to pursue this matter in some detail with the State Health Commissioner who presented overwhelming evidence that a voluntary immunization program would not be successful or worthwhile to maintain," and, therefore, he could not support our position. When I read that letter I couldn't help thinking, "What an admission! So the program can't stand on its own 'merits'; it has to be forced."

On November 15 I went to see Joe Canada, one of our state senators, to inquire about introducing an amendment to the compulsory immunization law to allow for an exemption based upon personal belief. He suggested that I would be wise to be satisfied with a "study" for the next year or two, because if I tried to push the bill through this time it would very likely be defeated. This bill will be tough to pass, he pointed out, because the law has been in effect for so long. He explained to me some of the convolutions of the legislative process and how even the simplest, most obviously needed legislation takes two and sometimes three years to get enacted.

At our January/1983 Health Federation meeting I spoke on "The Four Myths of Vaccination", and at our February meeting we showed the video tape, "DPT: Vaccine Roulette." Ellen Jacobs (not her real name), a teacher of natural childbirth, brought her class to both meetings. She told of two women she knew who lived in this area whose babies had died the very night after receiving their first DPT shot. Another person told of a friend of hers whose child died the night after receiving the DPT shot. Ellen also told of receiving a recent phone call from a former student of hers whose five-month-old baby girl had died one week after receiving the DPT shot. "The baby was breast fed and the parents were really into nutrition, too," Ellen said. In all these cases, the doctors denied any connection between the shot and the death. "What else could they do?" I pointed out. "If they admit a connection, they could not only be sued but their license and practice threatened."

During the course of the four years since the last court hearing, I have received many phone calls from parents who were determined not to have their child immunized and wanted to know how to avoid it. Many had an older child who had been immunized and had suffered various side effects, some apparently permanent. For instance, one mother who knew better let her son be immunized for admittance to school. He went into anaphylactic shock. She was determined that her younger child would never be immunized even if she had to keep her out of school. Another mother told how her baby girl became paralyzed on the left side after her third DPT shot. The child, who was seven at the time the mother talked to me, had a stiff left hand and a slight speech defect. Another mother who had a healthy six-year-old daughter who suddenly came down with rheumatoid arthritis remembered that she had let her daughter be immunized for German measles a month earlier. With the exception of the shock case, the doctors, as usual, denied any connection between the shot and the disability.

In many cases of a vaccine-injured child, the parent was opposed to, or at least hesitant about, immunizations but let herself be pressured into consenting. There is a bond between mother and child that is particularly strong during those early years, and any anxiety or resentment the parent feels can be picked up by the child. Surely there is a connection, no matter how subtle, between parental objection to a procedure and the child's subsequent negative reaction to it. After all, we are not decapitated bodies anymore than we are disembodied minds.

When doctors speak of "herd immunity" they use the same terms we use to describe cattle or sheep. They forget that humans are mental and emotional individuals as well as anatomical and biochemical ones.* We might say that mass, compulsory immunization programs treat not only fictional, standardized, textbook bodies, but headless ones as well.

During these same four years, I have been surprised to discover the subterfuges people use to protect their children from the immunization steamroller. I won't describe these because I don't want to jeopardize the only escape routes many people know.

When a woman from Pennsylvania called and wanted information on immunizations as well as how to avoid them, I looked at my list of exempt states and said, "Oh, you don't have anything to worry about. Pennsylvania is one of the free states." Afterwards I thought, "Hmmmmmmm . . . free and slave, terms used to describe states over one hundred years ago. We even have an 'underground railroad', parents—and doctors, I might add—who use subterfuges."

POWER AND PRIVILEGE SPEAK

On April 7, 1983, I phoned Joe Canada to enquire about the bill. He said he couldn't get enough support for the bill but would try to have

*For an excellent discussion of this point, see *You Are Extraordinary* by Roger J. Williams, Ph.D., Pyramid Books, New York, 1974.

hearings on it between now and January 1984. I told him I would give him some literature on the subject. A few days later I dropped off a copy of an early draft of Chapter 2 of this book as well as copies of some articles.

On May 6, 1983, the *Virginian-Pilot* came out with a front-page article titled, "Schools will require students to show proof of shots this fall." "Pupils not immunized to be barred" was the title of an article that had appeared in the *Ledger-Star* the previous day. The articles stated that there was a new and tougher immunization law passed by the General Assembly in 1982! The new law required, for instance, that private schools and day care centers must comply and that students' records must be checked for the exact dates of immunizations. A vice principal interviewed in a later article said he could get fined $10,000 for admitting a student who hadn't complied with the law. The articles did mention, however, the medical and religious exemptions.

By August, headlines were reading "Thousands of students still need shots," and "Tidewater schools bar 3,700." Various articles told of deluged clinics, vaccine shortages and borrowings from other cities, and harried personnel. I was interviewed as president of the local chapter of the National Health Federation and Tanya's case was mentioned.

I went to the library to get a copy of the tougher new law. Sure enough, the legislature had amended the section pertaining to the medical exemption. The law now said that the certification by a licensed physician would have to specify "the specific nature and probable duration of the medical condition or circumstance that contraindicates immunization." Another interesting amendment to the law was inserted into the first paragraph of the section on immunization requirements: "Neither this Commonwealth nor any school or admitting official shall be liable in damages to any person for complying with this section." What more is there to say?

UPDATE

Our chapter is no longer active. Two of our most dynamic and effective supporters, the vice president and the publicity chairperson, moved out of state. The energy that kept the chapter alive gradually dissipated. I, for one, had the growing realization that real change in a society comes about not by legislation, but by education. Passing a law when the consciousness of a critical mass of people does not accord with the law would be a holding action at best. The big issue here was not immunization, per se, but freedom of choice. The consciousness that is capable of grasping what this really means is a consciousness that understands that reality is relationships, that man is a spiritual being with the divine right to choose, and that truth is essentially harmonizing and liberating.

A society can change its direction only when a critical mass of people are capable of apprehending a larger truth, of seeing a larger vision. A few lectures on immunization won't do it. The scientific aspects alone are too much for a simple public lecture. No, a book was required.

This was even more emphatically brought home to me when I took a trip to Arizona recently. I gave a public lecture on immunization—"Immunization: Miracle or Myth?"—and met with a group of people who were working with the immunization issue there. Arizona is one of the more recent states to become "free," to exempt students from the vaccination requirement on the basis of personal belief. Yet, I was told, the schools and the media were ignoring the law, telling parents that it was a "no shots, no school" situation. Furthermore, parents told of children who were in school with the vaccine waiver but were forced to stay home and miss many important school activities, including, in some cases, graduation activities. They were excluded because the board of health declared an emergency—an epidemic. Where the evidence was for this epidemic is anybody's guess. As we have learned in Chapter 3, epidemics are not difficult to manufacture.

While I was there, a number of people on different occasions told me what I had heard before: There is constant pressure to get the personal belief exemption in the compulsory vaccination law rescinded. The pressure comes from the health department and behind it, the federal government. I was reminded of an elderly woman who attended a couple of our Health Federation meetings. Many years ago—I believe it was in the sixties—she and others had worked very hard to get the personal belief exemption clause inserted into the vaccination law in Virginia, only to have it rescinded shortly afterwards. (She, incidentally, was a registered nurse whose healthy baby daughter became cross-eyed shortly after her DPT shot.)

The story I have told here is an old story, one that has been repeated over and over throughout human history and is now being repeated daily, hourly upon this planet. It is the story of coercion, of power using privilege to impose "benefits" upon those who do not want them. It is the story of egotism, greed, and blind belief. Without the last, the imposition of these "benefits" on a large scale would be impossible. Liberating ourselves from the nursery of non-think in which blind belief flourishes is to begin the journey, not only to freedom, but to maturity.

11

■

WAKING
FROM THE PROPAGANDA
TRANCE

What luck for the rulers that men do not think!
ADOLPH HITLER

Ralph, what did you do today? Think or believe?
RALPH NADER'S FATHER

SNOW JOB PREVENTION

How do we keep from being duped and doped? Is there some way we can become immune to the vast epidemics of mindlessness that perennially sweep through our society? A good place to begin is to take a second look at "what everybody knows." Begin to ask questions: How do I know this? From what source am I getting my information? From what point of view is this idea true? From what point of view is it not true? As Alfred Korzybski, Polish engineer, mathematician, and founder of General Semantics used to say, "Whatever it is, it also isn't."

If an idea is presented as *the* explanation for some event or *the* solution to some problem, say to yourself, "That is one explanation. There are others," or "That is one solution. There are others." Try playing with other explanations which will lead to other solutions such

156

as reversing cause-effect relationships. When you read about scientists looking for a virus that causes a disease, say to yourself, "Maybe we should look for the disease that causes the virus." (Or better yet, "Maybe we should look for the condition that causes the virus.")

When you read or hear statements such as "doctors say" or "experts agree," the implication is that *all* doctors say or *all* experts agree. Say to yourself, "Have you interviewed every doctor—or expert—in the world?" Likewise, talk back to the expressions "nobody knows," "no known cure," and "no evidence for." Say to yourself, "Nobody you know knows," or "There is no cure you know of," or "There is no evidence you know about."

We are speaking, of course, of the proverbial sweeping or glittering generality, familiar to students of advertising and propaganda. General Semantics refers to these expressions as allness statements because they imply that someone knows everything about something. Try substituting "someness" for "allness" and say to yourself, "Some doctors agree" or "Some scientists say." Be alert for words like all, everybody, no one, no, never, always, entirely, totally, completely, and absolutely. They frequently signal an allness statement.

These little exercises are simple but subtle. They open rather than close the mind which, in turn, can lead to inquiry and discovery. As a number of people have observed, great contributions are made not by people who know the answers, but by people who know how to ask questions. The art of asking questions is largely the art of uncovering and challenging the assumptions hidden in our habitual patterns of thinking.

GOING SANE

Are language habits a pivot that can balance or unbalance the mind? Can we become "unsane" (Korzybski's term) by being ignorant of the nature and disciplined use of language? Can understanding the nature of language and using it in a disciplined, conscious way contribute to one's health and maturity?

In 1933, Korzybski published a ground-breaking book, *Science and Sanity*, which, in essence, answered the above questions in the affirmative. His book originated the science of General Semantics, which is the study of symbols—and words are symbols—and how we use and react to them. Man, as a symbol-using creature immersed in a world of symbols, can become "unsane" when he misuses them or reacts to them inappropriately. While most of the theory and principles of General

Semantics are beyond the scope of this discussion, a look at some of the principles should be enough to keep us from being mesmerized by many of the messages the mainstream culture sends to us.

The Non-Allness Principle we just discussed, for example, points to the idea that "no one knows everything about anything" because not only is human cognition and sense perception limited, but language, or any symbol system for that matter, is reductionist. The details of any given event that we choose to perceive and communicate are abstracted from an infinite number of possible details. Hence, interpretations are idiosyncratic —personal and peculiar to the observer-participant.

The allness statement has many faces. Can you recognize the allness statement in these two examples? "The most perfect man who has ever entered the Kingdom of Science."[1] This is an example of the unqualified superlative and was spoken by the great British physician, Sir William Osler. He was referring to Louis Pasteur. The Salk vaccine has been hailed as "the most dramatic breakthrough of the 20th century."[2] Here, the unqualified superlatives assume that the speaker is familiar with (1) all the scientists who ever lived, or (2) all the breakthroughs of the 20th century. The statements also assume that a purely objective standard of superiority exists. This doesn't mean that we shouldn't use superlatives. It would be difficult to express strong feeling without them. It does mean we should qualify our superlatives. Instead of saying "the greatest" or "the most" we should preface our statements with qualifiers such as "as far as I know" or "the greatest scientist I ever knew." This simple reminder that our viewpoint is only one of many, helps to promote humility, openness, and flexibility.

"Watch when you feel depressed," a friend of mine, psychologist, author, and teacher of General Semantics, Gina Cerminara, used to say. "If you'll watch closely, you'll find you are thinking in allness terms [e.g. I *never* do *anything* right or *no one* cares about me.] Allness statements box us in." Applying the Non-Allness Principle will contribute not only to mental health, my friend used to point out, but it will help us to become more tolerant and less precedent-bound. We will begin to ask, "Why am I doing this?" Then we will begin to examine some of the assumptions that have shaped our lives and open the door to alternative explanations and solutions.

One of the most pervasive and deeply embedded assumptions in our society—and probably most human societies—is the idea that some people have the right to tell other people what to do. These people have that right because they have greater knowledge or skills of a certain kind than the rest of us. How do they get that knowledge, what does it mean, and why do most people acquiesce to their pronouncements?

THE AUTHORITY MYSTIQUE

Pronouncements by experts—frequently representatives of established professional organizations—are another source of propaganda. When we see this appeal to authority we need to ask, "How do you know? What original research have you done? Are there vested interests behind your position?"

Who really is an expert? How does one become one? The term itself implies allness—someone who knows everything about something. If we look closely, we will discover that an expert is usually a person who has passed through certain academic rituals and has learned to see a segment of reality from a certain perspective. He has also learned to communicate ideas as seen from that perspective in a certain code or form of rhetoric. The limitations of a perspective can be disguised by exotic rhetoric.

What about the perspective of most medical doctors? They are probably the only group of experts whose orders we are enjoined to follow—"doctor's orders"—and whose pronouncements on the cause and treatment of disease are almost sacrosanct. This enormous amount of power and privilege blinds most of them—and most of us—to the obvious fact that their knowledge, like the knowledge of the rest of us, is limited and represents only one way of seeing and interpreting a set of data.

Some limitations of the medical (or allopathic) perspective are these:

(1) In medical school the focus of study is a cadaver, a dead body. Hence, the vital processes and energy patterns of a living body are lost, and the student tends to think of the body in static, mechanistic terms.

(2) The focus is on dissection and analysis of tissue; the relationship of the parts to the whole, therefore, tends to be lost. These limitations of perspective—which apply also to number 3 below—are camouflaged by esoteric language, the Greek and Latinate terminology used by the medical profession. This is part of the distancing process that creates the "authority mystique" of the professional. In my more impertinent moments, I have said that a medical education is largely learning some skills and a stance and dressing them in exotic nomenclature.

(3) Perhaps the most crucial limitation of the medical perspective is the built-in assumption that disease is an enemy that must be fought with weapons, i.e., drugs and vaccines. A number of writers have pointed out that medical schools in the United States are subsidized by the foundations and grants of the multi-billion dollar drug industry and that that same industry spends an average of $6,000 a year on every

doctor in the United States to get him to prescribe their drugs.[3] With a built-in bias like this, is it any wonder that the medical profession is disease rather than health oriented, and that we spend many times more money on health care than does Europe, England, Canada or Japan?[4] In fact, our total health care bill is now around $400 billion a year and is growing at a rate close to 15 percent annually.[5] As Linda Clark pointed out, "There is money in them thar' ills."[6]

Does this enormous expenditure buy better health? A cursory glance at a few statistics will dispel any notion that it does.* For example:

- 36 million Americans suffer from arthritis. 250,000 of these are children.[7]
- 12 million Americans have diabetes.[8]
- 43.5 million Americans have heart or blood vessel disease. 550,000 estimated to die of a heart attack in 1986.[9]
- 525,600 new cases of cancer are diagnosed yearly. 420,000 estimated to die of it in 1986.[10]
- More than two-thirds of all Americans suffer from chronic illness.[11]
- 132 million workdays are lost to illness at a cost to industry of $25 billion a year.[12]
- 40 to 60 percent of all disease complications in hospitals and clinics are iatrogenic (doctor induced).[13]
- 130,000 persons a year die from doctor prescribed drugs.[14]

The United States leads the world in the incidence of degenerative disease—and the consumption of refined food.[15] In 1979 we were pushing toward 40th place in national health among the community of nations.[16]

Is there any profession, other than the medical profession, where the disparity between cost and benefit is so great?

The maintenance of the authority mystique depends to a great extent upon limiting access to information and choices that challenge the position of the authority. Isolation is a well-known technique of brainwashing. Because the intellect learns by comparison, when it is presented with only one point of view or other points of view are denigrated, it loses its capacity to discriminate and ultimately its capacity for fully rational thought. We forget to our peril that there are many orders, degrees, levels, and kinds of realities which correspond to the

---

*As with any set of statistics the numbers vary according to the source. The figures I have here are on the conservative side. For instance, 40 million Americans (not 36 million) suffer from arthritis, according to Stephen M. Lindsey, M.D., a key speaker at a Health Fraud Conference in Virginia Beach (April 25, 1986).

many different minds that perceive and create those realities.* When we forget this we develop tunnel vision. We see only one way of doing or thinking about something. The remedy, of course, is this: Whenever you see only one way of doing or thinking about something, that is the time to look hardest for alternatives.

Anything perfectly obvious should, to some extent, be suspect. Nowhere, perhaps, is this better illustrated than in the myth of the objectivity of science and scientists. Not only is absolute objectivity an impossibility but scientists, being human, are emotionally and promotionally involved in what they are doing. So-called conflict-of-interest stories are by now proverbial. When a group in power has a vested interest in sickness, is it too much to suggest that their approaches to the solution of this problem will be as expensive, circuitous, and complex as possible?

But is medicine a science? Can anything that deals with so many unknown and uncontrollable variables be a science? "Physicians are not scientific in any meaningful sense. They get very technologic," Thomas Preston, M.D., reminds us.[17] When the primary subject of a field is as rich and resonant with ambiguities as a human being, we have moved into the realm of art. Isn't this why we refer to the field of healing as the healing arts, not the healing sciences?

HARDENING OF THE CATEGORIES

"A rose is a rose is a rose," goes the famous statement by Gertrude Stein. General Semantics would say, "Rose$_1$ is not rose$_2$ is not rose$_3$." Each is different and unique. We might say that a person who deals with people and objects in terms of their similarities and neglects their differences has "hardening of the categories." A more colloquial expression for this tendency is "lumpism," because the person with this tendency "lumps" certain people or ideas together into neat little categories, where they harden into stereotypes. That these stereotypes have little to do with reality can easily be illustrated by the example of a simple object such as a carrot. Carrots differ not only in size, shape, and color but in chemical composition and molecular arrangement. A

*Modern physics tells us that "this world does not exist in itself . . . (but) only as that met with by an ego." (Herman Weyl, *Mind and Nature*, University of Pennsylvania Press, Philadelphia, Pa., 1934, p. 1). Not only is the event dependent upon a mind (or ego) to give it reality, but mind shapes the event itself. The Heisenberg Uncertainty Principle states that the observer always interacts with the observed and the modes of perceiving alter the forms perceived.

carrot grown in one kind of soil will have different nutritive values than one grown in another kind of soil.

If such differences can be found among plants, think of the differences to be found among complex entities like human beings. Award-winning biochemist and professor emeritus, Roger Williams, points out in his book, *You Are Extraordinary*, how very different people are, not only anatomically but physiologically and biochemically as well.[18] On page 36, for instance, we see 12 pictures of "normal" livers each with a distinctively different size and shape. On page 34, we see 11 diagrams of the chemical constituents of the blood of 11 healthy young men. Each diagram is distinctly different, and each contrasts with the "textbook" diagram. In fact, as Dr. Williams points out throughout his book, the textbook standard is a fiction. So are words like average, typical, or normal. Each of us is unique.

This uniqueness extends to our minds and temperaments. We each have different life needs—for food, recreation, rest, stimulation, etc. One person might require 20 to 30 times more of a certain nutrient than another; a drug that might make one person drowsy would keep another awake. What is work for one person is play for another. Dr. Williams deplores the tendency to average people, to reduce them to a statistic, and warns that "we as individuals cannot be averaged with other people. Inborn individuality is a highly significant factor in all our lives—as inescapable as the fact that we are human."[19] To ignore the uniqueness of a human being is to ignore part of that very essence that makes him human.

What about mass, bureaucratically administered programs such as mass immunization programs? That the uniqueness of the individual tends to get lost in these programs is suggested by an article which appeared in the *International Medical Digest* (July 1969) which states: "There is no sound basis for the assumption that every child or infant must be inoculated with every available vaccine; on the contrary, there may be a valid reason for omitting any or all available antigens. Each patient is an individual, and deserves evaluation on this basis, rather than as an epidemiologic statistic." The article goes on to point out that "the incidence of vaccine-induced morbidity has increased alarmingly" and that the medical profession "must re-evaluate the principles, purposes, and hazards of immunization and reassess current procedures."[20] Assembly line medicine is bad medicine.

That mass vaccination programs create epidemics of non-think was eloquently expressed by Clinton Miller in his testimony against H.R. 10541 in the House of Representatives on May 17, 1962. After pointing to some of the problems with mass vaccination programs such as (1) serious side effects—e.g., encephalitis, coma, and death—suffered by some children, (2) little-known or publicized contraindications for vaccination, and (3) some statistical "hanky panky," Clinton Miller said:

> "In mass vaccination programs, it is common practice to omit or ignore such information in presenting the case for vaccination to the public. There is a tendency to let the "experts" make the decisions, after which they summarize the evidence with such press release statements as "absolutely safe," and other statements designed not to educate, but to inspire absolute confidence.
>
> "We point out that the tendency of a mass vaccination program is to "herd" people. People are not cattle or sheep. They should *not* be herded. A mass vaccination program carries a built-in temptation to oversimplify the problem, to exaggerate the benefits, to minimize or completely ignore the hazards, to discourage or silence scholarly, thoughtful and cautious opposition, to create an urgency where none exists, to whip up an enthusiasm among citizens that can carry with it the seeds of impatience, if not intolerance, to extend the concept of the police power of the state in quarantine far beyond its proper limitation, to assume simplicity when there is actually great complexity, to continue support of a vaccine long after it has been discredited, to make a choice between two or more equally good vaccines, and promote one at the expense of the other, and to ridicule honest and informed dissent."[21]

Just as people and objects are unique so are events. And, as with objects and people, the shared characteristics of any two events—or situations—are fewer than the differences between them. When a person wants to make a point by comparing these shared characteristics, we call this reasoning by analogy. Legal arguments that use precedents are using this kind of reasoning. Likewise, people who suggest a particular remedy for a current problem because a problem similar to it occurred many years ago and was apparently corrected by the recommended course of action are reasoning by analogy. People use this kind of reasoning when they point to epidemics that occurred many years ago and were apparently corrected by vaccination and warn that these same epidemics could occur now if there is fall off in immunizations. The problem with reasoning by analogy is again the problem of ignoring differences, some of which could be crucial. Certainly a past condition and a present condition are dissimilar in many important respects. We learned, for instance, in Chapter 4 that the conditions which created the epidemics of the past were very different from those that prevail in the civilized world today.

The use of faulty analogies to support an argument is common: Equating what happens in a test tube with what happens in a human body, for example, or equating humans with animals when supporting an argument for certain dietary practices. These observations and experiments have value, but they should be regarded as suggestive rather than prescriptive.

Post hoc reasoning which assumes a causal relationship between two events is also illustrated by the immunization example just discussed. Since this was discussed in Chapter 3, let's look now at the "Black and White Syndrome," or "Hardening of the Polarities."

HARDENING OF THE POLARITIES

To some, the world is divided into two camps—black and white, right and wrong. There is no middle ground, no gray, no alternative(s). This is the world of the person with, what I call, hardening of the polarities. General Semantics refers to this as either-or or two-valued thinking.

Two-valued thinking can be very useful for the propagandist because it creates false dilemmas. I once heard a pediatrician on television say that he explained to parents who were concerned about the dangers of vaccination that the risks of the disease outweighed the risks of the vaccination. He was saying in effect that there is only one way of preventing certain diseases, namely, immunization. He was also inferring that these diseases are irredeemable "bad guys" from which our children must be protected by medical technology. The propagandist creates the impression that there are only two solutions to a disastrous or potentially disastrous situation—his solution and the wrong solution. There are no alternatives.

CARD STACKING

This is really an extension of the two-valued thinking discussed above. The art of carefully selecting and presenting ideas and data—data which may or may not be true—so that only the best or worst possible case is presented is known as card stacking. There are no ambiguities; other possibilities are either ignored or discredited. The object is to get you, the reader or the viewer, to react strongly for or against an idea, an issue, a person, or an object. The pediatrician, just spoken of, buttressed his advice to parents by reminding the TV audience how immunizations wiped out—or nearly did—such dread diseases as smallpox and whooping cough. No credit was given to the contribution of such things as improved sanitation and personal hygiene, or the increased consumption of fresh fruits and vegetables. The detrimental side effects of immunization were barely mentioned.

Professor Gordon Stewart of Glasgow University remonstrates against this card stacking on the part of those who unreservedly recommend immunizations:

"What kind of immunisation is this for which success is being claimed? . . . What kind of epidemiology is this which advocates immunisation by excluding consideration of factors other than immunisation? . . . What kind of editorial policy is this which publishes incomplete data and promotes far reaching claims about the efficacy of immunisations but refuses to publish collateral data questioning this efficacy?[22]

Card stacking can be concealed by misleading use of words. For instance, a free newspaper bearing the masthead of one of the two leading newspapers in our community used to be delivered to our home every Wednesday. Opening the newspaper we found headlines on such medical topics as "Safe exercise OK during pregnancy, experts say" (May 22, 1985), and front-page articles on medical topics such as, "Nation marks 30th year free from the specter of polio" (April 17, 1985), or "'Remedies' for arthritis called fake" (May 9, 1985). From two-thirds to three-fourths of the articles were about medical "breakthroughs" and related topics such as medical advice and stories of people struggling with some disease or disability that is medically managed. Is this really a newspaper? I would call it medical advertising.

Misleading video pictures and discussions, where only the spokesmen for a particular group are present, are other examples of card stacking. For instance, I saw on television a segment of a news program that had been advertised earlier in the day as a "discussion on chiropractic." The discussion turned out to be a medical doctor telling the viewers that orthopedic care of serious back problems was more effective than chiropractic. He conceded that chiropractic was more effective for minor back problems, but only because the chiropractor, unlike the orthopedist, took time to discuss appropriate exercise and nutrition with his patient. At the beginning of this "news" segment the viewer was shown a picture of a patient lying face down on a chiropractic table being adjusted by a woman "chiropractor." The woman wore dark red lipstick and had long dark red fingernails. Need I say more?

LOADED WORDS AND PICTURES

Perhaps the easiest way to get people to do what you want them to do—and this is the goal of the advertiser and propagandist—is to stack the deck with loaded words and pictures, i.e., words and pictures with emotionally charged meanings or connotations. Referring to a disease as a "hidden menace" or a "killer and crippler" is an example of loaded language. The picture of chiropractor just described is an example of a loaded picture.

Whatever the picture of the "chiropractor" with long red fingernails suggests to you, it hardly suggests a health care professional who works primarily with her hands and fingers. To refer to an essentially benign, self-limited disease of childhood such as rubella or German measles as a "hidden menace" or a "killer and a crippler" is again using language to mislead. (No doubt, the writers were referring to the birth defects associated with rubella if contracted during the first trimester of pregnancy. But, as Dr. Moskowitz points out, vaccines for childhood diseases, such as measles, mumps, and rubella, can transform these essentially benign, self-limited diseases of childhood into their more serious counterpart in adolescents and young adults. Thus rubella vaccine can actually increase the risk of birth defects.)[23]

One of the best places to pick up obvious and sometimes colorful examples of loaded words and pictures is your local health department. The folders are replete with most of the propaganda devices we have been discussing: *post hoc* reasoning, misleading statistics (Chapter 3), glittering generalities, appeals to authority, lumpism, two-valued thinking, card stacking, and loaded words and pictures. Another excellent source is your local newspaper, particularly articles celebrating the life-saving virtues of some new vaccine or drug. In the literature from both these sources, words such as dread, devastating, deadly, strike, danger, risk, wipe out, etc., can usually be found, particularly at the beginning of the text. These are words calculated to get attention and arouse the reader, in this case, arouse fear and a subsequent dash to the doctor for protection.

What about a word like "quack"? It is a label usually applied by the medical establishment to either an alternate health care system (quackery) or a health care practitioner who uses unapproved therapies; its purpose is to convince the reader to go only to standard brand (medical) doctors who use standard brand therapies. The word "quack" is associated with incompetence and deception and suggests a person who pretends to have knowledge or skill he doesn't possess. The label is derogatory and loaded—really old-fashioned name-calling.

Loaded labels like other loaded words can mislead, but sometimes even more so, because labels are, in a sense, libels. When we label a person or a group we tend to imply allness. We throw a person or a group into a category and close the case. When we read of hear the word "incompetent" applied to someone or some group, we need to ask, "With respect to what?" Aren't we all incompetent with respect to something? Even relatively non-loaded labels, like honest and intelligent, when applied to someone, need to be questioned. Aren't we all honest or intelligent in some ways and in some circumstances and not in others?

Perhaps you have noticed that most of the propaganda techniques discussed are really different versions of the allness statement. The nature of language and the nature of human thinking tend toward generalizations. We couldn't communicate without them. We simply need to be aware that generalizing can be a trap. Overgeneralizing is, according to Stuart Chase, "probably the most seductive, and potentially the most dangerous, of all fallacies."[24]

Man's tendency to think that value can be measured in terms of popularity or consensus is, I think, part of this need to generalize. Let's look at a propaganda technique that exploits man's need to identify himself with a group.

BANDWAGON

A recent editorial in our local newspaper which argued for the passage of a law requiring the use of seat belts began by pointing out that 16 states now have this law and the use of seat belts is increasing. This is known as the bandwagon appeal, the appeal to join the crowd or be left out. The spokesperson for the health department who said that one half of one percent of the children eligible for vaccinations receive exemptions and 65,000 children were vaccinated in Virginia last year (Chapter 9) was suggesting that everybody's doing it so it must be right—bandwagon.

The idea that something is right or good if enough people are doing it is one of the most seductive of mental traps. We don't have to go back very far in history to find that much of what most people thought and did was not necessarily good or true. Perhaps the seductiveness of "others, therefore me" lies in our human need to belong, to be accepted. This is our strength and our weakness: Our strength in that our group consciousness can help us be more aware of the needs of others; our weakness when we become mindless conformists.

THE WORLD AS PROCESS

"We can never step into the same river twice," Heraclitus said. "The only constant is change." As the river changes from moment to moment, so does the world. The idea is obvious, yes, but easy to forget. We tend to assume, for instance, that the person we saw yesterday is the same person today, or that a particular magazine we read five years ago has the same editorial policy today. We forget that people and objects have a uniqueness in time as well as in space.

When we enter the microscopic and submicroscopic worlds of molecular and atomic energies, the world as process becomes more apparent. On this level, change is continuous and instantaneous; we can see ourselves and the universe as a process in space-time. On the level of ordinary reality, however, our senses record only gross differences that are apparent only with relatively long lapses of time. Subtle changes that occur from moment to moment usually escape us.

To illustrate the distortions of time and our senses my friend, who taught General Semantics, had her classes do some simple experiments. One experiment which was quite a source of merriment for the class, was to have each person at the end of a row whisper some simple message into the ear of his/her neighbor. The message was repeated in this way to each person in the row (about eight times). The person at the other end told the class what the message was. What that person said was such a distortion of what the first person had said that everybody laughed. When the experiment was repeated using a single message for the whole class—about thirty repetitions—the distortion was so great, the original message was almost unrecognizable.

Most of what we know of the world is based upon reports, and each report has been filtered through the motives, biases, and conditioning of different reporters. Even two people witnessing the same event will describe and interpret it differently, as the Japanese film "Roshomon" illustrated so well. My friend would illustrate this point for her class by holding up a drawing of a scene in a department store. After a few minutes she put the picture down and asked some questions about it. As you might guess, there were almost as many different answers as there were students in the class.

Do these experiments tell us something about the nature of language—and the nature of knowledge? For a starter, we might ask, "Is the noun or object centeredness of our language partly responsible for our tendency to regard processes as things?" We speak of diseases as though they were entities rather than processes. Microorganisms are labeled as though they were microentities rather than stages of an evolutionary cycle. A doctor frequently conducts tests to determine how a patient's disease "entity" can be labeled. Diagnosing and labeling disease entities is an important part of medical practice. A number of people have observed that this preoccupation tends to promote the treatment of labels, not disease processes, and certainly not people. Nowhere is this better illustrated than in mass immunization programs.

THE WORLD AS PROJECTION

"We see what we know," Goethe said. "It is our theories that determine what we see," Einstein reminds us.[25] We do not live in a world of hard facts, but a world of perceptions and interpretations. Believing is seeing. The microbial world, for instance, looks like this to some researchers:

> These microscopic biochemical components . . . constantly are at war between themselves and their external and internal environment.
>
> "Like the humans of which they are integral parts, they form and break alliances with each other. Some, following the pattern of international intrigue, act as double agents, scientists report.
>
> "In this never-ending battle, evolutionary changes constantly take place which enable the microscopic participants either to play more effective roles, or to become the slaves of more dominant factions, or even to be absorbed and become a part of them, research shows.[26]

Other researchers have seen molecular and bacterial interactions suggestive of cooperation, even self-sacrificing behavior.[27]

We project onto the world our beliefs and assumptions about it. General Semantics might put it this way: We abstract from an infinite number of details those that fit into our frame of reference.

Facts and values are mutually dependent. There is evidence, for instance, that the "objective" observations of scientists—as well as the theories they create and prove or disprove—reflect the subjectivity of the scientist as well as the value system of the society in which the science operates.

There is also evidence that human beings in a scientific investigation tend to behave in a manner consistent with the observer's theory. They respond to the expectations of the observer.[28] We know plants and animals respond to color and sound vibrations as well as human thought intention. We need to recognize ourselves in the world we see and interpret.

THE WORLD AS SYMBOLS

Man is an "amphibian"; he lives in two worlds—the world of physical reality and the world of symbols. The latter is supposed to communicate information about the former; however, as we have pointed out, it doesn't always do this. A primary reason it doesn't—and one we haven't discussed yet—is that we fail to check our verbal maps by going to the territory, to use Korzybski's terms. Languaging tends to get divorced from experiencing. Obviously we can't experience directly all our assumptions about the nature of the world. I assume England is there, but I am not going to go there to see if it is. I am going to rely on reports and reports of reports, etc.

We should be aware, however, that when we read a report we tend to assume its truthfulness. And that is the problem. Propaganda masquerades as news and information. For instance, I have a copy of a section of a university newsletter warning people about the hazards of raw milk and recommending pasteurization.[29] The article refers to studies to support its position but gives no specifics other than to mention the group (Centers for Disease Control) who conducted the studies, a group long associated with the position taken by the article. Advocates of the nutritional superiority of raw milk are given short shrift with expressions such as "no evidence" and "no way." The news is one-sided and deals in generalities—the essential coin of propaganda.

When we read a report of an experiment or a study, we should at least ask who funded it and where and when it took place. Technical and professional publications usually include a reference as to where more particulars such as size, duration, and controls can be found.

When we see a set of statistics, we might want to know how some of the figures were arrived at. Numbers can vary considerably from source to source. Conclusions and interpretations of the same studies and experiments can also vary from one researcher to another.

One of the most effective tools of the propagandist is to support an argument by comparing two or more groups of people and pointing out that only the group that has or does what he recommends shows the desired result. If we look closely, however, we will find that only one or two factors among many significant factors have been considered. The variables have not been controlled.

An article on heart disease, for instance, points out the flaws in some of the studies upon which a prestigious scientific group, the National Institutes of Health, bases its position.[30] The studies involve comparing several population groups. However, only two factors (amounts of saturated fats and cholesterol in the diet) among many significant factors were studied and a causal relationship attributed to these two factors. This particular scientific group has held the same position for many years; and, I suspect, they approach their research deductively— that is, they attempt to find more evidence to support a conclusion already formulated and hardened into official policy.

This is one of the problems with scientific research. Science pretends to be inductive, to search for answers by explaining facts and deriving principles from them. Too often, however, money and vested interests indicate the most profitable answers and fund scientists to search for evidence to support them. Thus, politics can masquerade as science.

BACK TO PRINCIPLE

If knowledge, as this entire discussion has suggested, is tenuous—and picking our way through a maze of propaganda and misinformation is tricky—is there some relatively simple and straightforward way we can recognize that which has genuine worth? I think there is. When confronted with two or more conflicting studies, claims, or systems of thought, ask yourself, "What is the operative principle behind this claim or system of thought?" Is it essentially negative or positive? That is, is it based upon preventing an undesirable condition or is it based upon creating a desired condition? Does it build upon fear and avoidance or upon harmonizing and connecting? If the former, the paradigm and the solutions suggested by it will be fragmented, out of context, and detail-ridden. If the latter, the paradigm and the solutions it suggests will be more holistic and free from a plethora of details.

We might say positive is beautiful. Surely the vision of a desired condition has more aesthetic potential than the vision of an undesired condition. So the other side of the coin of "back to principle" might be "back to beauty." As we pointed out in Chapter 8, the aesthetic criterion is a very valid one. We are drawn to the beautiful in other areas of life, why not scientific paradigms that are beautiful? Physicist, author, and distinguished historian of science, Thomas S. Kuhn, has written that there is "another sort of consideration that can lead scientists to reject an old paradigm in favor of a new. These are arguments, rarely made entirely explicit, that appeal to the individual's sense of the appropriate or the aesthetic . . . the importance of aesthetic considerations can sometimes be decisive.[31]

So when we must choose between two or more conflicting claims or systems of thought, why not choose the one that pleases us aesthetically? As Dr. Kuhn points out, scientists may do this. If this seems

TABLE 4. INDOCTRINATION *vs.* EDUCATION

INDOCTRINATION (PROPAGANDA)	EDUCATION
1. Uses generalizations, "allness" statements: Lacks specific references and data.	1. Uses qualifiers: Statements supported with specific references and data.
2. One sided: Different or opposing views are either ignored, misrepresented, underrepresented, or denigrated.	2. Circumspect and multi-faceted: Issues examined from many points of view. Opposition fairly represented.
3. Card stacking: Data carefully selected to present only the best or worst possible case. Language used to conceal.	3. Balanced: Presents representative samples from a wide range of available data on the subject. Language used to reveal.
4. Misleading use of statistics.	4. Statistical references qualified with respect to size, duration, criteria, controls, source, and subsidizer.
5. Lumpism: Ignores distinctions and subtle differences. Lumps superficially similar elements together. Reasons by analogy.	5. Discrimination: Points out differences and subtle distinctions. Uses analogies carefully, pointing out differences and nonapplicability.
6. False dilemma (either/or): There are only two solutions to the problem or two ways of viewing the issue—the "right way" (the writer or speaker's way) and the "wrong way" (any other way).	6. Alternatives: There are many ways of solving a problem or viewing an issue.
7. Appeals to authority: Statements by selected authority figures used to clinch an argument. "Only the 'expert' knows."	7. Appeals to reason: Statements by authority figures used to stimulate thought and discussion. "Experts" seldom agree.

TABLE 4. Continued

INDOCTRINATION (PROPAGANDA)	EDUCATION
8. Appeals to consensus (bandwagon): "Everybody's doing it" so it must be right.	8. Appeals to fact and logic: Supports arguments with impartially selected data and logic.
9. Appeals to emotions and automatic responses: Uses words and pictures with strong emotional connotations.	9. Appeals to people's capacity for thoughtful, reasoned responses: Uses emotionally neutral words and illustrations.
10. Labeling: Uses labels and derogatory terms to describe proponents of opposing viewpoint.	10. Avoids labels and derogatory language: Addresses the argument, not the people supporting a particular viewpoint.
11. Ignores assumptions and built-in biases.	11. Explores assumptions and built-in biases.
12. Language usage promotes lack of awareness—unconsciousness.	12. Language usage promotes greater awareness—consciousness.

capricious because ideas of beauty are subject to personal bias, what isn't subject to this bias? Surely the paradigm that points in the direction of greater freedom, holism, and harmony is more beautiful than one that points in the direction of dependency, fragmentation, and alienation. On a practical level, this means that the natural would take precedence over the artificial, the whole would take precedence over the part, and self-help would take precedence over institutionalized help.

But then, this is my bias. Yours may be something else, hence the need for choice.

NOTES

1. Sir William Osler, "Introduction," *The Life of Pasteur*, Rene Vallery-Radot. Quoted by J. I. Rodale, "Bechamp or Pasteur?", *Prevention*, Aug. 1956, p. 71.

2. Marcia Dunn, "Nation marks 30th year free from specter of polio," the *Virginian-Pilot*/EXTRA, April 17, 1985, p. 2.

3. Maureen Salaman, *Nutrition: The Cancer Answer*, Statford Publishing, Menlo Park, Calif., 1984, p. 10. Robert S. Mendelsohn, M.D., *Confessions of a Medical Heretic*, Contemporary Books, Chicago, 1979, p. 36.

4. Dan Rather, CBS Evening News, Dec. 6, 1985 (statement on Europe and England); "Health Notes," *Health Freedom News*, Feb. 1985, p. 38 (statement on Canada and Japan).

5. Betty Kamen, Ph.D., "Notes from the Establishment," *Health Freedom News*, Jan. 1986, p. 17.

6. Linda Clark, *Get Well Naturally*, ARC Books, New York, 1972, p. 16.

7. Arthritis Foundation, Jan. 1986.

8. News broadcast, Nov. 30, 1985.

9. American Heart Association, 1985 Heart Facts Reference Sheet.

10. Linus Pauling Institute of Science and Medicine, Palo Alto, Calif., 1986.

11. Paavo Airola, *Everywoman's Book*, Health Plus, Phoenix, Ariz., 1979, p. 30.

12. John McManus, "Wellness Center: 'A Way of Life,' " *Ledger-Star*, May 31, 1982.

13. Leonard Jacobs, "Menage," *East/West Journal*, Sept. 1977.

14. Maureen Salaman, "Homeopathy: the personalized natural therapy," *Public Scrutiny*, July-Aug. 1981, p. 30.

15. Howard Fugate, M.D., address at Oak Tree Country Club in Pennsylvania, reported by Bill and Irma Ahola in *Shaklee Newsletter*, Dec. 1982.

16. *Organic Consumer Report*, May 15, 1979.

17. Thomas Preston, M.D., Donahue Show, Jan. 7, 1982, Virginia Beach, Va.

18. Roger J. Williams, *You Are Extraordinary*, Pyramid Books, New York, 1974.

19. Ibid. p. 17.

20. Airola, op. cit., p. 289.

21. Hearings on H.R. 10541, May 16, 1962, p. 86.

22. Gordon Stewart, M.D., *British Medical Journal*, Jan. 31, 1976, reprinted in *The Australasian Nurses Journal* by Drs. Kettman and Kalokerinos, "'Mumps' the word but you have yet another vaccine deficiency," June 1981, p. 17.

23. Richard Moskowitz, M.D., *The Case Against Immunizations*, reprinted from the *Journal of the American Institute of Homeopathy*, vol. 76, March 1983, page 19.

24. Quoted in *You Are Extraordinary*, p. 193.
25. Quoted in *The Healing Continuum*, Patricia Anne Randolph Flynn, Bowie, Md., Robert J. Brady Co., 1980. Quotes are from Introduction.
26. Julian DeVries, medical editor, *Arizona Republic*, March 29, 1976. Reprinted by William A. McGarey, M.D., "Medical Research Bulletin," *Pathways to Health*, Aug./Sept. 1979, Phoenix, Ariz.
27. Marilyn Ferguson, *The Aquarian Conspiracy*, J. P. Tarcher, Los Angeles, Calif., 1980, p. 165.
28. George S. Howard, "The Role of Values in the Science of Psychology," *American Psychologist*, March 1985.
29. Tufts University Diet and Nutrition Letter, "News from the World of Medicine," *Reader's Digest*, April 1985.
30. Ruth Adams, "Is Cholesterol the Villain?" *Better Nutrition*, May 1985, pp. 26–28.
31. Thomas S. Kuhn, *The Structure of Scientific Revolutions*, University of Chicago Press, Chicago, 1970, pp. 155–56.

SUGGESTED ADDITIONAL READING

1. Gina Cerminara, *Insights for the Age of Aquarius*, Prentice-Hall, Englewood Cliffs, N.J., 1973.
2. W. Ward Fearnside and William B. Holther, *Fallacy—The Counterfeit of Argument*, Prentice-Hall, Englewood Cliffs, N.J., 1959.
3. "How to Say What You Mean," *Nation's Business*, May 1957.

12

■

THE COMING
REVOLUTION IN
HEALTH CARE

Man was created for the sake of choice.

HEBREW SAYING

FROM EITHER/OR TO
MULTIPLE OPTION[1]

"All progress has to do with increasing choices and options. If you talk about one society being more progressive than another, you talk about a society in which citizens have a greater freedom and greater range of choices and possibilities," Nathaniel Brandon, author and psychologist, told his audience. He pointed out how biological and evolutionary development is founded upon the increase of options and choices. "If you talk about progress in the biological or evolutionary sense from an amoeba up to man, you're looking at organisms with increasing variability of response. They are able to do more and more things in response to the environment. The range of possibility keeps growing. If you think of people who do bodywork, any kind of opening of the body, working

176

with blocks, whether it be Rolfing or any of the other types of work, it is always to make it possible for the body to do more things. If you think of psychotherapy, where a person we say is stuck or rigid. What do we call progress? It always has to do with increasing the ranges of choices and options."[2]

Options and choices will be central to the health care system of tomorrow. Choice is essential, not only to the health of a democratic society, but to the health of the person as a whole. Knowing that we have choice empowers us, makes us feel responsible for our condition, and augments our impulse to participate in both our own healing and the healing of our society. There is "overwhelming evidence that the mind is a key controlling factor (if not *the* key controlling factor) in virtually all disease," Edgar Mitchell, former astronaut and founder of the Institute of Noetic Sciences, tells us.[3] To deny choice is to deny the role of the mind in the healing process. In fact, recent research "assures that any medicine that ignores the power of the conscious mind will ultimately be declared unethical."[4]

We are moving from a society with few choices to one of many— either/or to multiple options, according to John Naisbitt (*Megatrends*). What does this mean with respect to health care? We will see more growth in the alternative health care fields such as physiotherapy, homeopathy, naturopathy, herbology, chiropractic, acupuncture, and midwifery. A recent newspaper article discussed the impending doctor glut and the steady decline in the demand for physicians while nonmedical health care specialists are experiencing a boom cycle. Compared with 1960, for instance, by the year 2,000 the number of chiropractors and nurse-midwives is expected to triple.[5]

The result of a national poll in which over 50 percent of the respondents said they would seek treatments rejected by the medical community if they were stricken by serious disease was reported in another recent article. In the same poll, 50 percent of the respondents approved of allowing clinics to operate in the United States that treat cancer and other diseases in ways opposed by mainstream medicine.[6] This is remarkable considering the vigorous propaganda of the medical establishment damning "unproven" remedies and the near blackout of positive reportage on these remedies—which generally offer no profit for drug companies.

Are we witnessing the beginnings of the dissolution of the great American medicine show? Certainly, increasing numbers of Americans are becoming disenchanted with the institution of disease scare, symptom management, and complicating side effects, not to mention the skyrocketing price tag. More Americans are beginning to suspect that much of the literature emanating from authoritarian institutions such as the medical establishment is possibly propaganda. We as a people are outgrowing authoritarian institutions and their style of relating, a style assumed by people whose assumptions about human nature and the natural world are negative and narrow. If the future belongs to democracy—and I think it does—it belongs to those people and those institutions whose assumptions about the nature of themselves and their world are essentially benign and life-affirming. What could be more life-affirming than the assumption that men are essentially good and capable of deciding what is best for themselves? This, of course, is the assumption behind the democratic ideal and the founding documents of this country. When enough people can open themselves to develop democratically, that is, become freer, less obstructed and less attached to authority—titles and precedents—we will have a democratic society.

It is already happening. Health care practices are well into reflecting Naisbitt's megatrends six and eight—movements from institutional help to self-help, and from hierarchies to networking.

FROM INSTITUTIONAL HELP
TO SELF-HELP

Television actress Linda Evans told a packed audience in the Senate Hearing Room how she had overcome severe allergies with the help of a nutritional counselor after she had been unsuccessfully treated with dangerous drugs like cortisone.[7] Thousands of people, including myself, could tell similar stories, stories of healing a chronic ailment by changing eating habits and otherwise adopting a more healthful lifestyle. In my own case, which I mentioned in Chapter 4, I took courses from doctors who used natural methods of healing; I read books and was counseled by others who were knowledgeable in these methods. Like Linda Evans, I, too, first went the conventional medical route. My childhood days were punctuated by regular visits to the allergy specialist for shots. The result: The hayfever of my childhood became the asthma of my later adolescence and early adulthood.

Be Your Own Doctor is the title of a book by nutritionist and naturopath Ann Wigmore. "Everyone over forty should be his own doctor," Dr. Jensen used to say. Presumably it takes that long to learn how to live healthfully. The idea of being our own doctor—except for serious accidents—has been echoed by many other health care practitioners. Learn how to live and forget doctors, they say. Megatrend number six (from institutional help to self-help) suggests that this may indeed be the wave of the future.

FROM HIERARCHIES TO NETWORKING

"The new health care model will be people helping people," Roger Jahnke, multidisciplinary health care practitioner, told his class. "We need to be health care practitioners for each other."[8] Since this was a class in body therapies—neuromuscular release facilitated by working with partners and using such modalities as reflexology, bodywork, and acupressure—this statement was particularly apropos. We are the only culture—and this is true of industrial cultures generally—that depends upon experts for health care, he said. In earlier cultures, people took care of each other.

What then is the role of the expert? Increasingly, I think, we are going to turn to the expert or medical specialist only for crisis situations, such as mechanical and chemical accidents, and to ourselves and to each other for health maintenance and working with chronic ailments. The health care professional will become more of a teacher and counselor and only secondarily a dispenser of pills and potions. The holism that was lost during the Middle Ages will return, and the practitioner will not only work with the patient as a mental, spiritual, and physical being but will himself be a spiritually conscious person. Assembly-line health care—treating labels and symptoms—will be confined to crisis situations.

I look forward to the day when the philosopher-physician, like Plato's philosopher-king, will be the ideal, if not the norm. This is a person so spiritually attuned that knowledge, virtue, and love are fused. Knowledge of this caliber is experientially derived insight into the values and principles embedded in the very structure of the universe.

At the least, we will expect a health care practitioner to be an example of health and to have a "healing presence." As we move from the model of physician as technician and symptom manager to the model of physician as teacher and healer, those health care professionals who are skilled in working with their hands, such as body therapists, chiropractors, and acupuncturists, will be in greater demand. Because many of these skills—for example, massage, polarity, shiatsu, acupressure and bodywork—do not require large investments of time and money to learn, we will see more people becoming skilled practitioners of these healing arts. As we learn to help ourselves and each other by sharing knowledge and skills, healing will become democratized.

FROM SHORT-TERM TO LONG-TERM

Expedient or quick-fix solutions that create long-term damage are losing ground to less expedient, long-term solutions. When we talk about long-term solutions we are talking about those that involve whole systems rather than parts of systems. The quick-fix solution seeks to isolate and alter a part. The long-term solution works with wholes—whole systems and whole persons. In an interview with Peter Barry Chowka, Dr. Michael Smith, who uses herbs and acupuncture to treat drug addicts, said, "Pharmacological science always seeks to alter just one thing—a bacteria or a nerve, for example. The drug is supposed to have this single effect; although in practice, it always has twenty other effects— side effects. The whole process is totally separate from the way life works."[9] From the short-term to the long-term—from the part to the whole—is the trend away from treating effects towards removing causes.

"Art is simple, but art is long," a music teacher friend of mine used to say. Substitute the word "healing" for the word "art" and we have the essence of natural healing and the new paradigm shift in health care. As disillusion with symptom-treating, technological medicine increases, we will see more people opting for the simpler but more long-range solutions of natural and holistic healing.

No discussion of long-term solutions would be complete without mentioning agriculture, because many of the principles that apply to creating health in humans—and animals—apply to creating health in plants. Healthy plants, like healthy humans, do not attract pests nor are they susceptible to diseases. Many experiments have demonstrated that plants grown on organically mineralized and balanced soil do not attract pests nor do they get diseases as do plants grown on deficient and chemically fertilized soil.

One example among hundreds that could be cited is described by horticulturist Sand Mueller: "I had read claims by organic gardeners saying their healthy plants had no insect problems. I believed these assertions were preposterous, as did every horticulturist I knew." He then describes how the bug problem in his garden completely disappeared after using compost. His first composted garden coincided with a year of cutworms. The cutworms were everywhere—except in his garden.

His second composted garden coincided with the year of the locusts. Swarms of grasshoppers severely damaged the alfalfa in the surrounding fields before coming to his garden. "For five days they buzzed around my lettuce, tomatoes, beans, peppers, and cabbages. Then they all left," he tells us. Although every part of the garden was swarming with grasshoppers, the only damage they did was to eat five small cabbages. In a quarter of an acre of tender garden plants, not a single leaf, other than the five cabbages, was damaged and he had used no poisons of any kind.[10]

A number of studies have shown that insects can detect subtle mineral imbalances in plants and devour only those plants that are out of balance. "Satellite photographs of Africa have shown how gigantic flights of locusts will cover thousands of miles ignoring healthy vegetation, then descending and destroying fields where the soil is worn out."[11] Again we see that pests, like bacteria, are nature's undertakers, returning the unfit to the elements for recycling.

Over a hundred years ago, the great pathologist Rudolf Virchow said that "germs seek their natural habitat—diseased tissues—rather than being the cause of the diseased tissue; e.g., mosquitos seek the stagnant water, but do not cause the pool to become stagnant."[12] With Kirlian photography and other energy measuring devices we now know that the cells of every form of life—plant, animal, human, and microorganismic—emit radio signals as well as photons (light).[13] A strong, healthy plant radiates wavelengths of a different frequency from that of an imbalanced, unhealthy one. Strong, virile plants—nurtured in soils mineralized and rich in humus—"broadcast" wavelengths harmless to humans and animals, but which act like a protective screen against pests.*[14]

Poisoning crops with pesticides is a bit like driving a car and shooting the oil gauge when the red light goes on. We're treating an effect, an indicator. As our understanding of ecology and the interdependence of all life increases, these shortsighted solutions will wane. We will seek life-enhancing solutions that work with whole systems, not isolated parts. We will respect all forms of life, knowing that each in some way contributes to the welfare of the whole.

FROM MASS TO ENERGY

Instead of going to the doctor for physical exams and check ups, will we go for "energy field studies"? We know that sickness shows up in the energy field before it shows up in the physical body, and early detection shortens and simplifies therapy. "Gradually, human anatomy

---

*Another way of interpreting this might be that balanced and unbalanced plant cells emit different signals, which are detected by insects. Could we infer that something similar happens on a human level?

will be recognized as energy anatomy, and physiology as energy physiology, when medicine catches up with physics," Harvey Grady, director of the John E. Fetzer Energy Medicine Research Institute, points out.[15]

As we move from an object-oriented consciousness to an energy-oriented consciousness, we will think of the body more in terms of energy fields than of a composite of physical and biochemical parts. Actually, noninvasive electrodiagnostic and therapeutic techniques are being used now. Europe has been using electrodiagnosis for 20 years and we in the United States are using low frequency electro- and electromagnetic therapy for pain relief, to restore the function of paralyzed or weakened nerves or muscles, and to accelerate the healing of cataracts and other ailments. Electromagnetic currents have also been used to regenerate limbs; grow severed nerve cells; and accelerate repair of skin ulcers, wounds, and bone fractures in rats and salamanders. "Many ancient civilizations used energies in sophisticated forms of healing, such as Chinese acupuncture 5,000 years ago," Dr. William McGarey reminds us. "Now is the time to reclaim that heritage."[16] Part of reclaiming that heritage will be learning to utilize therapeutically the energies of sound (including music), light (including color), and heat, as well as the more subtle energies of thought, feeling, and visualization.

Energy balance and imbalance on a cellular level seem to be the primary signifiers of health and disease states. Electrodiagnosis uses very sensitive instruments to detect energy imbalances as they manifest in various organs of the body. Energy therapies seek to redress these imbalances. Are we returning to earlier researchers such as Bechamp, Rife, Koch, and Warburg who told us that disease begins in unbalanced cell metabolism which, of course, reflects some kind of unbalancing influence in the life of the host organism? And isn't the transition from an object-centered consciousness to an energy-centered consciousness an aspect of the transformation from fragmentation to holism and from isolation to connectedness? For it is on the level of energy—information-bearing energy, electricity, consciousness—that we are whole and connected and that our mind-body is one.

FROM SUBSTITUTION TO REGENERATION

"Plato said, more than two thousand years ago, that what is honoured in a country, will be cultivated there," warned the Executive Board of the World Health Organization. "We may have to take a second look at what we honour."[17]

The evening news features an item on the progress of the latest heart transplant recipient; the local newspaper tells a heart rending story of a child who needs a liver transplant; a popular magazine tells the story of the heroic boy who saves the life of his brother by giving him his healthy kidney. The story of the man who regenerates his heart by diet, herbs, cleansing, exercise, etc., is not news, neither is the story of the child who regenerates a failing body by a change in life style. Enlightened self-discipline is not the stuff of high drama. It is also not the stuff of large investments in expensive technology. In short, it is not the stuff of big money and our cultural penchant for magic and melodrama.

As our disease care system grows more expensive and inefficient, and as our awareness of the pressing needs of the larger global community grows, we are going to ask ourselves some searching questions such as: Does the enormous expense of high tech, high drama disease care, which at best can benefit a very few, justify itself? How can we transform expensive disease care into cost-efficient health care? How can we reorient our thinking to move from doctor dependency to self-reliance, and from drug and surgical intervention to self-regulation and organ regeneration?

RECYCLING DINOSAURS

"B Complex, Inositol—Nature's Tranquilizers."
"Herbal Formula Helps Regenerate Pancreas"
"Aluminum, Fluoride Implicated in Alzheimer's"

Headlines of the future? When the trends toward self-care and networking, holistic and ecological thinking, and long-term solutions that are simple and harmless reach a critical mass, we will see headlines such as these. When the trend toward multiple options reaches a critical mass, we will read articles in the popular press about the research and discoveries of natural schools of healing such as herbology, homeopathy, chiropractic, etc. And when the current peace movement becomes perceptive enough to see that peace begins in consciousness and in the language that reflects that consciousness, then the healing of our planet, our language, and ourselves will begin. Bellicose rhetoric such as "battle of the budget" and "keeping the democratic knives from cutting too deeply," typical of the rhetoric of politics, will be replaced by metaphors suggesting connection and cooperation.

"The future exists in language," Werner Erhard told his audience.

TABLE 5. HEALTH CARE MODELS

OLD OUTER-DIRECTED DISEASE CARE	NEW INNER-DIRECTED HEALTH CARE
1. Palliative: Emphasis on removing symptoms. Aims for quick results.	1. Educative: Emphasis on removing causes through knowledge and its integration into living habits. Aims for long-term results.
2. Authoritarian: Emphasis on management and control. Professional "manages" disease; patient "follows doctor's orders."	2. Egalitarian: Emphasis on patient participation and recovery. Professional gives guidelines; patient directs his own therapy.
3. Assembly-line methods geared for profit.	3. Client-centered methods geared for autonomy.
4. Relies on technological intervention and substitution, e.g., organ transplants, insulin injections, synthetic and frequently toxic drugs, immunizations. Focuses on replacing organs or their functions.	4. Relies on harmless, noninvasive therapies and substances, e.g., food—including herbs and supplements; water—used both internally and externally; visualization; body movement and alignment. Focuses on regenerating organs and restoring their functions.
5. Cost and dependency escalating.	5. Cost and dependency de-escalating.
6. Disease and disability seen in terms of victimization and melodrama.	6. Disease and disability seen as self-created and preventable, the natural consequences of violating principles.
7. Mechanistic: Body seen as mass, an object containing discrete parts.	7. Organic: Body seen as energy, living patterns, and interacting fields.
8. Fragmented: Body and mind treated separately. Parts of body regarded separately and treated singly.	8. Holistic: Body-mind treated as a unity. Parts of body treated in relation to other parts and aspects of the body-mind.

TABLE 5. Continued

OLD OUTER-DIRECTED DISEASE CARE	NEW INNER-DIRECTED HEALTH CARE
9. Atavistic: Disease seen as entity separate from patient.	9. Contemporary: Disease seen as process, inseparable from patient.
10. Adversarial: Disease seen as enemy.	10. Unifying: Disease seen as corrective.
11. Externalizes causality: Focus is outside the patient: viruses, bacteria, poisons, and stresses in the environment.	11. Internalizes causality: Focus is on the patient: his choices, attitudes, habits, and reactions to environmental influences.
12. Disease oriented: Focuses on labeling and controlling or destroying disease entities. Research focuses on prevention and elimination of disease. Absence of disease seen as the result of technological intervention.	12. Health oriented: Focuses on supporting the natural healing energies of the patient. Research focuses on what creates optimum health. Absence of disease seen as by-product of health.
13. Uses military rhetoric: "building defenses," "fighting," "battle against," "strike," "attack," "weapon," etc.	13. Language suggests harmony and cooperation such as referring to disease as a healer, and detoxification as a cleanser.
14. Monolithic and coercive.	14. Pluralistic and voluntary (multi-optioned).
15. Negative: Builds on fear and distrust of the natural world. A system of "disease-scare."	15. Positive: Builds on rapport and cooperation with the natural world. A system of health care.

"Where being shows up is in language."[18] Linguistic violence reflects mental violence which becomes physical violence. A harmonious consciousness reflects itself in peace-oriented language. Here we must begin if we would have healing for ourselves and our planet.

How can we recycle the military metaphors of the medical model to suggest an ecological and essentially harmonious relationship with microorganisms and the health and disease processes to which they are related? What metaphors can we use that will suggest harmony, interdependence and stewardship rather than conflict, alienation, and victimization? What metaphors will help us to think of our bodies as extensions of our consciousness and the world around and within them as a continuum of life support systems?

We might begin by referring to our illnesses as a reaping of imbalances or unwise choices instead of something that "strikes" us or that "bug going around." Instead of saying, "I caught a cold," why not say, "I created a cold."? This helps us to be aware that we are responsible, empowered beings. Louis Pasteur used to refer to the "invaded patient." I suggest we use the term "client" rather than "patient" because it connotes working with rather than working upon—a partnership rather than a paternal or administering relationship. And, of course, we are not invaded; we create conditions that produce consequences.

The military metaphors describing the immune system and its functions need to be recycled to suggest an ecological system within a larger ecological system, instead of a battlefield within a larger battlefield. Instead of terms such as "building defenses," "building resistance," and "conquering disease," we could use terms such as "enhancing health," "creating harmony," and "cleansing and balancing." These terms are more bland and don't pack the adrenal charge as do the old metaphors. Perhaps, someone with a more poetic gift than mine will come along and give us metaphors that are more incisive and dramatic.

What about the word "immune"? My medical dictionary says the word immune comes from the Latin *immunis* which means "safe." My Latin-English dictionary says it means "with no public obligations, untaxed, free from office, exempt, free from." Is this the metaphor we want to describe a system that is capable of rendering foreign substances harmless or possibly transforming them into something the body can use? A metaphor whose focus is on being safe or free from some burden or threat?

I remember a TV program, "The Body in Question," in which we saw a leucocyte (white blood cell) surround and devour a foreign object. The narrator, Dr. Jonathan Miller, told us that white blood cells are nature's garbage collectors. So instead of white blood cells being warriors and first lines of defense they were clean-up crews. They clear out morbid or toxic matter. Why not have a name that suggests cleanliness or honors the capacity of cells to transform their environment and in turn be transformed by it? What about a name like "the transform system"? Or, if we want to be more elegant and Latinate, we could call it the "mutationis system," which means a system that exchanges and alters. Pretentious, yes, but more positive and dynamic than *immunis*.

Once we begin using more affirmative metaphors, the idea of injecting poisons into one's body for the purpose of "building defenses" to "fight disease" becomes ludicrous. I predict the time will come, perhaps in our lifetime, when the administration of toxins—drugs and vaccines—either for the prevention or treatment of disease will be looked upon much as we now look upon the practice of bloodletting. Doctors will attempt to justify the practice of vaccination long after it has been discredited. However, the justification for the practice of vaccination will be particularly tenacious, because another element has entered the picture: unlike the old practitioners of bloodletting, the vaccinators have gone to the government and enlisted its powers to enforce obedience to their dogma.

What about the term "preventive medicine"? Both words need recycling. When we think in terms of prevention, we focus energy on preventing an undesirable condition instead of creating a desirable condition. What we give energy to expands. Do we want to expand more undesirable conditions and more ways to prevent them? What about the term "medicine"? To most of us it suggests using something unpleasant to get rid of something bad. How can we change this negative into a positive? If our goal is the creation and enhancement of health, why not call our health care program simply that—a health care program?

But more importantly, the term "medicine" has been overdone in our culture. It has been used to refer to a system of health care that has too long monopolized the health care market. Medical research, medical science, medical advice, medical authority, and medical supervision are terms we use automatically as though the medical model were some kind of absolute—the way things are. Using other terms such as health research or health care supervision might help to open us to the possibilities of other models, other approaches.

Once we begin to recycle language, our fascination with pathology and its classification will yield to a more holistic perception of the relationship between health and disease. "Disease is nothing but life under altered conditions," pathologist Rudolf Virchow reminds us. And it is conditions which should be the object of therapy, not diseases, he adds.[19] The myriad possibilities of the whole, the healthy, the optimal, and the conditions which produce them will be the occupation of the health care system of tomorrow.

What about recycling some of the more destructive elements of the medical-pharmaceutical and agrichemical industries? How can these industries be retooled to produce biologically and ecologically supportive commodities such as compost, organically grown food, natural and organic food supplements, ecologically supportive energy sources, and training for health-oriented health care practitioners? We could extend this redirection, of course, to include other businesses such as the food processing business, the media, and the military.

When the adversarial consciousness and the language habits that feed it are recycled, the destructive elements within the social institutions of a culture also will be recycled. Form follows consciousness.

FULL CIRCLE

> *The universe, like a bellows,*
> *Is always emptying, always full. . . .*
>
> *"Life and death, though stemming from each other, seem*
> *to conflict as stages of change. . . .*
>
> LAOTZU, *Tao Teh Ching*

The idea of the universe as a bellows and life and death as complementary cycles of a larger whole recurs perennially throughout religious, philosophical, and mythical literature. From the days and nights of Brahman to the yin and yang of Taoism, man intuited that the universe was a living entity with cycles of inhalation and exhalation, expansion and contraction, growth and decay, creation and dissolution. Now physics is discovering that pulsation, a dynamic expansion and contraction, is indeed the core of all experience.[20] On the human level, we are rediscovering that good health depends upon balancing these forces—the anabolic and the catabolic—within the body.* Emanuel Revici, M.D., has, for instance developed a system of medicine utilizing these concepts and has had remarkable success using it in treating seriously ill patients.[21]

Have we forgotten something, man has known intuitively for thousands of years? In our fixation on dissection and analysis, we see fragments—opposition where there is complementarity, dissolution where there is cleansing, death where there is renewal. Shiva, the third member of the Hindu trinity, represents the aspect of destruction or dissolution and is recognized by the Hindus as part of the life process. (The other two aspects of God are Brahma and Vishnu, the creator and preserver.) Because our inclinations and our instruments predispose us to see only

---

*In this context, anabolic refers to processes that are constructive and proliferative, and catabolic to processes that involve the liberation of energy and the utilization of stored resources.

one-half of the cycle, we fear the other half; that half we see darkly. And so we fight it.

"From the most primitive life forms, viruses and bacteria, to the most evolved body cells in the cerebrum, our bodies include a constantly evolving continuum of life forms," writes Leonard Jacobs in his explication of the macrobiotic point of view. "The primitive forms are not our enemies, but constitute the evolutionary origin of our body cells and the eventual future of our bodies returning to the soil in the grave."[22]

Substituting microzymas (small ferments) for viruses and bacteria in the above quotation, we get a simplified idea of what is meant by the phrase "ecology of the body." We could think of disease symptoms as the body's attempt to rebalance an internal ecology that has become imbalanced through unwise choices and living habits. "Perhaps one day our medical schools will start paying due attention to the person, realizing that the human being is the only reality, and that disease is born out of the malfunctioning life that dwells within that individual," Dr. William McGarey tells us.[23] As we have seen, that malfunctioning life resonates on many levels.

What will future historians call our age, an age when people used the same short-sighted application of technology to pollute their bodies as they did to pollute their planet, an age when the body and its infirmities were exploited for profit, an age when the fascination with and fear of pathology reached epic proportions (witness the current AIDS hysteria), an age when the earth and its resources were treated as if they were insensible and infinitely expendable commodities, an age when the universe and most of its life forms were seen as hostile and people fought diseases as they fought each other?

Currently, we are enmeshed in a nuclear dilemma whose resolution, according to Jonathan Schell, can occur only when we "reinvent the world."[24] When our vision becomes whole—healed—and our ecological awakening includes the mental and microscopic universes, we will graduate from the model of a mechanical, mindless, threatening universe into a model of a living and loving one. Then the mentality of attack and defend will be outgrown, and we will have reinvented the world.

NOTES

1. John Naisbitt, *Megatrends*, Warner Books, New York, 1984. See table of contents and text for this and other megatrends discussed in this chapter.

2. Nathaniel Branden, Ph.D., talk recorded in Del Mar, Calif. 1981, by Mandala Outer Circle, untitled.
3. Letter by Edgar D. Mitchell to members of the Institute of Noetic Sciences.
4. Background of leaders and description of course given at Omega Institute, July 26–27, 1986, p. 37 of Catalog. Leaders are: Jeanne Achterberg, Ph.D., G. Frank Lawlis, Ph.D., Michael Harner, Ph.D., and Lawrence LeShan, Ph.D.
5. Don Colburn, "Doctor supply outpaces nation's growth," *Washington Post News Service*, reprinted by the *Ledger-Star*/EXTRA, Dec. 12, 1985.
6. Lawrence Kilman, "Permit unproven cancer clinics to operate, 50% say in survey," *Ledger-Star*, Feb. 6, 1986.
7. Clinton Ray Miller, "The Washington Report," *Health Freedom News*, Jan. 1986, p. 27.
8. Roger Jahnke, Workshop and Lecture on Body Therapies, Association for Research and Enlightenment, Virginia Beach, Va., May 10, 1983.
9. Peter Barry Chowka, "The Organized Drugging of America," *Health Freedom News*, Oct. 1983, p. 9.
10. Sand Mueller, "A Horticulturist Speaks Out on Health," *Health Science*, April/May 1980, pp. 27–31.
11. Ibid. p. 28.
12. American Natural Hygiene Society, Inc., (Bulletin), July 7, 1955, p. 32.
13. *Brain/Mind Bulletin*, Aug. 19, 1985, "Living cells emit light, German scientist reports," p. 1.
14. *Organic Consumer Report*, Topanga, Calif., Jan. 26, 1982.
15. *Pathways to Health*, The A.R.E. Clinic, Phoenix, Ariz., Sept. 1984, p. 1.
16. Ibid.
17. *Organic Consumer Report*, Topanga, Calif., Dec. 14, 1976.
18. Werner Erhard, "Taking a Stand for the Future," cassette tape, 1983.
19. Rudolf Virchow, quoted by Karl Menninger, *The Vital Balance*, Viking Press, New York, 1963, p. 41 (book written with Martin Mayman and Paul Pruyser).
20. "Movement psychology: freeing 'postural beliefs,' " *Brain/Mind Bulletin*, April 18, 1983, p. 1 (idea is from psychologist, Stuart Heller).
21. "Emanuel Revici: Evolution of Genius," *Impact*, Spring 1985, special supplement.

22. Leonard Jacobs, "Menage," *East/West Journal*, Sept. 1977, p. 14.
23. William McGarey, M.D., "Medical Research Bulletin," *Pathways to Health*, Phoenix, Ariz., June 1985, p. ii.
24. Johnathan Schell, *The Fate of the Earth*, quoted by Willis Harman, "Hope for the Earth, Connecting Our Social, Spiritual and Ecological Visions," Institute of Noetic Sciences, Fall 1982, p. 1.

SUGGESTED ADDITIONAL READING

1. Gavin Borg, "Sounds Foretell Disease," *Moneysworth*, Winter 1986.
2. William Campbell Douglass, M.D., "Employee Health and The Tomato Effect," *Health Freedom News*, Feb. 1986.
3. "Germanium—Element #32," *Organic Consumer Report*, Topanga, Calif., June 14, 1983.
4. Don Matchan, "Hierarchy Halts Treatment of Cataract With Low-Pulse Energy," *National Health Federation Bulletin*, Oct. 1980, pp. 22–24.
5. "Radionics—By Any Other Name," *Organic Consumer Report*, Topanga, Calif., July 29, 1980.
6. "What's in a Name?", *Organic Consumer Report*, Topanga, Calif., July 23, 1985.

PART IV

■

APPENDIXES

APPENDIX A

■

KEYS TO A HEALTHY
IMMUNE SYSTEM
(A Holistic Approach)

I. PHYSICAL
  A. Keep the body alkaline by:
    1. Eating plenty of fresh fruits and vegetables. For most people the proportion should be 80 percent alkaline-forming food to 20 percent acid-forming food. In general, fresh fruits and vegetables are alkaline forming and starches and proteins are acid forming. The more physically active a person is, the more acid-forming foods his body can handle.
    2. Eating only whole, natural foods. As much as possible eat food that is fresh, in season, organically and locally grown, with an emphasis on green leafy vegetables.* Eat most food raw or slightly steamed.
    3. Chewing food well; saliva alkalinizes food.
    4. Eating whole grains that have been germinated. Germination makes them more alkaline, easier to digest, and increases protein and enzyme content.
    5. Keeping eliminative organs working well and periodically going on short cleansing regimes.**
    6. Getting adequate rest, exercise, pure water, and fresh air.

*Some writers and therapists, such as those of the macrobiotic and Natural Hygiene school of thought, maintain that childhood diseases can be avoided by eliminating dairy products (in the context of a health-promoting life style, of course). I suspect that it isn't the elimination of dairy products per se that produces results, but the elimination of the adulterated dairy products—pasteurized, homogenized, chemicalized—that are consumed.
**A cleansing regime consists of certain dietary restrictions along with bowel cleansing, exercise, rest, pure water, and fresh air. The dietary restrictions consist primarily of eliminating concentrated proteins and starches and living on fresh fruits and vegetables and/or their juices. The duration is usually from one to eleven days.

195

B. Avoid:
   1. Refined sugar.
   2. Refined, chemicalized, stale, and overcooked food.
   3. Poisons such as drugs, vaccines, insecticides, x-rays, radioactivity.
   4. And, of course, coffee, tobacco, and alcohol.
C. Take supplements as needed. The following nutrients specifically support the immune system:
   1. Vitamins C, A, E, and the B complex.
   2. Minerals zinc, calcium, magnesium, iodine, iron, and selenium.
   3. Herbs such as garlic, alfalfa, echinacea, yarrow, ginger root, cayenne, and *taheebo.**
   4. Lemons, acidophilus culture (for colon).

For more information on dosage and preparation of herbs, see the following references:

Paavo Airola, *Everywoman's Book*, Health Plus, Phoenix, Ariz., 1979.

John Christopher, *Childhood Diseases*, Christopher Publications, Springville, Utah, 1978.

Jethro Kloss, *Back to Eden*, Longview Publishing House, Coalmont, Tenn. 1950.

Barry Sultanoff, M.D., "How to Strengthen Your Immune System," *East/West Journal*, Jan. 1986.

II. MENTAL
  A. Practice:
    1. Moderation: Do nothing in excess.
    2. Positive thinking: Give energy to the desired condition.
    3. Open-mindedness: Believe you can have the desired condition.
    4. Visualization: See the desired condition.
    5. Balanced living: Balance physical, mental, social, and spiritual activities.
  B. Avoid:
    1. Reacting negatively or stressfully to a situation.

III. SPIRITUAL
  A. Practice:
    1. Seeing yourself as part of an "unbroken wholeness," in which every part supports every part.

---

*Special mention should be made of the remarkable herb, *pau d'arco* or *taheebo*, from the bark of a South American tree. Unlike most medicinal herbs, *taheebo* is eminently palatable. A delicious tea that can be given to children is made by simmering the bark and adding a little peppermint tea and/or honey.

2. Seeing the universe as harmonious and life-affirming.
3. Seeing your body as an energy field, an extension of your consciousness which responds to your thoughts and feelings.
4. "Centering" and getting in touch with your transpersonal self and its life-affirming energies.

APPENDIX B

■

HOW TO AVOID IMMUNIZATIONS LEGALLY

If you do not want your child vaccinated, what should you do? Virtually all states have a compulsory immunization law requiring children to be immunized against certain childhood diseases: diphtheria, pertussis, tetanus, measles, mumps, rubella, and polio. Failure to comply with the law can prevent your child from attending school and expose you to possible criminal penalties.

First, read the law. You will find there are two and sometimes three exemptions: medical, religious, and personal belief. To qualify for the medical exemption you must have a doctor certify in writing that vaccines would be detrimental to your child's health. To qualify for the religious exemption a parent or a guardian must sign a notarized affidavit stating that immunizations conflict with the child's religious beliefs. If your state is one with the personal belief exemption, simply write on a piece of paper that immunizations are contrary to your beliefs. The following states have, as of 1985, the personal belief exemption: Arizona, California, Colorado, Idaho, Indiana, Iowa, Louisiana, Maine, Michigan, Minnesota, Missouri, Montana, Nebraska, North Dakota, Ohio, Oklahoma, Pennsylvania, Rhode Island, Utah, Vermont, Washington, and Wisconsin.

If your state does not have the personal belief exemption and you cannot get a medical exemption, the easiest course for you to follow would be to take the religious exemption.

"It is possible for parents to file as conscientious objectors with the state health department although this choice is not advertised," Carol Horowitz tells us. She says that several people she knows who are conscientious objectors state that it is their "God-given right to refuse to immunize my child." Any lesser statement is legally unacceptable. You cannot say, for instance, that you have read 20 articles in newspapers and 8 articles in medical journals or have seen some documentary on television.[1]

In his book, *Dangers of Compulsory Immunizations/How to Avoid*

Them Legally, attorney Tom Finn describes some legal tactics that may be used but do require the services of a lawyer. If you wish to pursue this course you may want to obtain his book. Write Family Fitness Press, Box 1658, New Port Richey, Fl. 33552. Certainly, compulsory immunization laws raise constitutional issues such as the violation of the First, Ninth, and Fourteenth Amendments as well as violation of civil tort law.

How to Legally Avoid Unwanted Immunizations of All Kinds, a booklet published by the Humanitarian Publishing Company in Pennsylvania, is another good source of information on avoiding immunizations. You can obtain it by writing the Humanitarian Publishing Company, R.D.3, Clymer Road, Quakertown, Pa. 18951.

What about traveling abroad? You simply declare exemption under Clause 83 of the International Sanitary Code, issued by the World Health Organization and adopted by all its members. It states, in effect, that only when coming from an infected area are vaccinations necessary *or* the traveler could be quarantined for up to 14 days from the time he left the infected area *if* the health department deems it necessary. If you come from an area where there has been an epidemic, you will probably be put under surveillance. This simply means that together with the local health officer you must keep a close watch for any suspicious signs or symptoms. You will probably be required to report periodically to your local health officer for a period of up to 14 days from the time of your departure from the infected area. If you notice any outbreak or symptom, you must immediately turn yourself in and submit to quarantine or isolation.

In actual practice this possibility is very remote: and if it should occur, the vaccinated person may be required to submit to the same surveillance as the unvaccinated! Remember, every year thousands of unimmunized tourists travel in and out of the United States with little or no inconvenience or embarrassment.

For more information and guidance on immunizations, contact the National Health Federation, P.O. Box 688, Monrovia, Calif. 91016. Phone: (818) 357-2181. For more information and guidance regarding immunization of school-age children, including exemption letters based on state laws, contact The American Natural Hygiene Society, 12816 Racetrack Road, Tampa, Fla. 33625.

NOTE

1. Carol Horowitz, "Immunizations and Informed Consent," *Mothering*, Winter 1983, p. 38.

APPENDIX C

■

SOME NATURAL REMEDIES FOR CHILDREN'S AILMENTS

The following information was obtained from a local nurse-midwife who has worked for two pediatricians who used nutritional therapy. By following these "rules," she told me, her own children have never been ill for more than one day.

Rule No. 1: If child is sick take him off dairy and flour products. Of course, nothing made with white sugar is ever permissible.

Rule No. 2: Give child large doses of vitamin C with pantothenic acid and calcium.

Rule No. 3: Keep the bowels open with either an enema or an herbal bowel cleanser such as Herb-Lax.

Rule No. 4: If possible fast the child and give him/her teas such as camomile, catnip, fennel, peppermint, etc.

For a sick child in general: Diet of green beans, celery, zucchini (Bieler Broth). Broth is made by steaming the above vegetables and liquefying them.

For diarrhea: Brown rice and steamed carrots. For small child, liquify.

For colds: Fasting and vitamin C. One thousand mg. of vitamin C for every year up to age ten. The addition of pantothenic acid makes this therapy even more effective. If the child is very young and whines for food give him/her some fresh fruit.

For general mucus conditions such as earache, bronchitis, sinus, etc.: Give child fresh fruits and vegetables, chicken, and peanut butter. (Can fill celery sticks with peanut butter) No dairy products and no flour products.

To these general remedies herbalists might add lemon, garlic, capsicum, alfalfa, and high doses of vitamins A and C for both prevention and treatment of infectious diseases. Besides the books mentioned in Appendix A, there are a number of excellent books outlining naturopathic and herbal remedies for specific ailments.
Here are some we have found particularly helpful:

1. Henry G. Bieler, M.D., *Food is Your Best Medicine*, Random House, New York, 1969.
2. Louise Tenney, *Today's Herbal Health*, Woodland Books, P.O. Box 1422, Provo, Utah, 1983
3. Michael Tierra, C.A., N.D., *The Way of Herbs*, Unity Press, Santa Cruz, Calif., 1980.

Nothing said here, of course, is meant to substitute for consultation with a health care professional who is knowledgeable in natural methods of healing.

APPENDIX D

■

INSTEAD OF SUGAR

Because refined sugar consumption weakens the immune system and has been implicated in a number of serious diseases such as cancer and mental illness,[1] we should replace this non-food with real food. A "sweet tooth" is generally indicative of a vitamin B deficiency; the craving for sweets usually disappears when adequate amounts of a natural source of vitamin B complex, such as nutritional yeast, are taken. Nature provides an abundance of fruits to satisfy our need for sweets, so when we need a sweetener or something sweet why not try the following:

Fruits and Fruit Concentrates

Fruit concentrates using fruits such as pear, pineapple, grape, and peach juices are now being used by a number of producers of natural foods to sweeten drinks, cookies, cereals, candy bars, and even chocolate sauce. In our family we usually use apple juice as a sweetener for lemonade and for the iced herb teas we drink in the summer. We use about ½ herb tea to ½ apple juice.

For popsicles, dissolve 1 tablespoon of gelatin in a scant ¼ cup cold water. When softened, add about ¼ cup boiling water and stir until dissolved. Add this mixture to about 1½ pints of unsweetened fruit juice such as pineapple, orange, or grape. Beat in blender, pour into popsicle molds, and put in freezer.

Fruit juice sweetened syrups are available and make delicious toppings for cereals, pancakes, and ice cream. Date sugar, made of dehydrated, pulverized dates, makes a good sweetener for baking as do raisins and currants. These more concentrated sweeteners should generally be used in colder weather when we need more concentrated foods.

Grain Sweeteners

Barley malt, rice syrup, and amazake. Although expensive, one of the advantages of these newer sweeteners is that they are composed largely of maltose which is released into the blood more slowly than the sugars of other natural sweeteners which are largely sucrose and fructose. This helps to stabilize the blood sugar.

Maple Syrup and Blackstrap Molasses

Maple syrup is regarded by many as the premier gourmet sweetener among natural sweeteners. Although less processed and more expensive than blackstrap molasses, it, like blackstrap, does require boiling to produce. Unlike other sweeteners, molasses has a strong flavor which can limit its use.[2]

Honey

Of all natural sweeteners other than fresh fruit, honey—natural, raw, unheated, unfiltered, unprocessed—is the only one that could be called a medicinal food. Pollen-rich honey, Dr. Airola tells us: (1) increases calcium retention; (2) increases hemoglobin count, thus preventing or curing nutritional anemia; (3) is beneficial in kidney and liver disorders, colds, poor circulation and complexion disorders; (4) has a beneficial effect on healing processes in such conditions as arthritis, constipation, poor circulation, weak heart, and insomnia; and (5) retards aging. In one study of longevity Russian biologist Dr. Nicolai Tsitsin found that a large number of centenarians were bee keepers and all of the centenarians, without exception, said their principle food was honey![3]

So we see that $sugar_1$ is not the same as $sugar_2$ which is not the same as $sugar_3$. The chart comparing the difference in the way our bodies handle refined white table sugar and unrefined, raw, unfiltered honey illustrates this point. We could even construct a chart comparing different natural honeys. Generally, the darker the honey the richer it is in minerals.

To substitute honey for sugar in cooking, use ¾ cup honey for every cup of sugar and reduce other liquids by ⅕. Ice cream is probably the easiest dessert to make with honey. Use the same recipe as for making popsicles, substituting top milk (unhomogenized, of course) for fruit juice and use from ⅓ to ½ cup of honey and 2 teaspoons of vanilla. For "chocolate" ice cream I use carob powder, and for fruit and nut flavors I use natural fruits and nut flavors. To make the ice cream richer I add several tablespoons of skim milk powder (noninstant). My daughter, Ingri, makes a delicious ice cream using lecithin granules instead of gelatin. Her recipe is this:

In a blender mix in order the following: 2 eggs, 1 cup cream, 3 heaping tablespoons lecithin granules, 2 teaspoons pure vanilla, ½ cup honey, 1 cup cream. To make a full quart, add a bit more milk-cream

COMPARATIVE NUTRITIONAL VALUES
OF SUGAR AND HONEY

SUGAR*	HONEY**
acid reacting	alkaline reacting
supports bacterial growth	kills bacteria
oxidizes or burns intensely in the body producing a shock effect on the nervous system and vital organs	gradual and even absorption by the body
intense stimulation followed by a slump	no letdown
addictive	contains built-in satiety factor, self-limiting
drug-like effect	food
empty calories—leeches vitamins and minerals (particularly calcium and vitamin B_1) from the tissues to metabolize itself	contains vitamins, enzymes, minerals, utilized by the body as a food
primary cause of many diseases such as poliomyelitis, diabetes, arthritis, heart disease, ulcers	has been used to prevent and treat certain diseases such as polio, diabetes, arthritis
stimulating	relaxing and mildly sedative
contributes to constipation	mildly laxative
forms toxic metabolites such as pyruvic acid and abnormal sugars containing 5 carbon atoms which interfere with cell respiration in the brain, blood, and nervous system	burns clean—no toxic metabolic residue

*Sugar refers to refined, white, table sugar (sucrose).
**Honey refers to raw, unfiltered, unpolluted (no chemical additives) honey.
SOURCES: *Sugar Blues*, William Dufty, Warner Books, New York, 1975.
     Honey and Your Health, Bodog F. Beck, M.D., Bantam Books, New York, 1971.
     Sweet and Dangerous, John Yudkin, M.D., Bantam Books, New York, 1973.
     Diet Prevents Polio, Benjamin P. Sandler, M.D., The Lee Foundation For Nutritional Research, 1951.
     "The Use of Honey in the Prevention of Polio," D.C. Jarvis, M.D., *American Bee Journal*, Aug. 1951, pp. 336–37.

and pour into freezing trays. When frozen, cut mixture into strips and homogenize in the Champion Juicer. Serve with ground almonds. To make the ice cream less mucus forming and to give it a delicious maple flavor, add three tablespoonsful of slippery elm powder and eliminate the eggs (I use one egg).

Because obtaining quality milk and cream—unpasteurized and un-homogenized—is very difficult if not impossible for most people in the United States, many health-minded consumers are substituting nut and seed milks. We make a delicious ice cream using sesame seed milk. To a quart of sesame seed milk add about three heaping tablespoons of lecithin granules, two teaspoons vanilla, and about 1/2 cup honey. Blend in liquefier. Pour in ice tray and place in freezer. When frozen, put cubes through the Champion Juicer. To store, put in plastic containers and place in freezer.

To make nut or seed milks, simply blend about ¼ cup raw nuts or seeds—almonds, sesame, cashews—with a cup of water in a liquefier and add one or two tablespoons of honey or maple syrup. Blend until smooth—usually three or four minutes at high speed. To make milk richer, increase quantity of nuts or seeds. To make milk smoother, strain through a cheesecloth or fine strainer. Also, soaking nuts or seeds overnight helps to make the milk smoother and easier to liquify. The skins of almonds can easily be pulled off after they have been soaked overnight, thereby producing a sweeter, whiter milk, (Hulled sesame seeds also produce a sweeter, whiter milk.) To blanch almonds before soaking them, simply boil water and immerse the almonds in it for thirty seconds. The skins will come off easily.

We prefer to use apple juice as a sweetener, so we substitute ½ apple juice for ½ of the water. We also like a richer milk, so we use ½ cup seeds or nuts to 1½ cups liquid. Double this recipe for a quart of ice cream and liquify about 8 or 10 minutes.

Flavors, of course, can be varied. For almond or lemon flavor add 1 teaspoon almond or lemon extract. Different fruits and fruit juices, such as banana or pineapple, can be added. With a little imagination you can make a variety of delicious, non-mucus forming ice cream.

To make malts, put cubes of frozen ice cream mixture in a blender with enough milk to cover blades. Blend and eat. If the cubes are vanilla flavored, you can add carob or fruit to the milk to vary the flavor.

Here is our favorite cookie recipe, excellent for cold weather and so simple my seven-year-old grandson can practically make these cook-ies himself: In a fairly large bowl mix the following ingredients: ⅔ cup oil (cold pressed—we use olive oil); ⅔ cup honey; 1 egg; 2 teaspoons lemon flavoring; ½ teaspoon cinnamon; ¼ cup whole wheat flour; ½ cup *fresh* wheat germ or a mixture of soy flour, bran, and protein powder; 1 teaspoon salt; 3 cups rolled oats; 1 cup sunflower seeds; 1 cup raisins. If batter is too dry, add a bit of water. Drop by teaspoons onto greased cookie sheets and bake at 325° for 15 to 20 minutes.

Making candy with honey is simplicity itself. The basic recipe is this: Mix together equal parts of honey, nut butter, milk powder (non-instant), nuts and seeds. Roll in wax paper, put in freezer, and slice when frozen; or press into flat oiled trays, put in refrigerator, and cut into squares. Here is my daughter's favorite candy which she calls "Super Fudge": Use equal parts of honey, peanut butter (smooth), and carob powder. Add chopped walnuts and/or sunflower seeds and enough shredded coconut (unsweetened) to make a thick consistency. Either roll in wax paper, put in freezer, and slice when frozen; or shape into balls, roll in coconut, and put in refrigerator.

Mental Imagery

Ever tried cutting carrots crosswise and calling them carrot cookies? Or slicing apples crosswise, coring them, and calling them apple doughnuts? Or cutting celery into three inch pieces, filling the groove with peanut butter, and calling them celery boats? A little imagination can turn an ordinary vegetable into a gourmet adventure. It can even turn disaster into triumph. For instance, my daughter recently made a super cake with all natural ingredients. It didn't rise. She forgot to put in baking powder. It was like the "rock of Gibraltar" so we called it "Rock Cake" and ate every chip.

The foregoing suggestions are just a few of the ways you can transform health-destroying sugar addiction into conscious choices that support health.

NOTES

1. A number of researchers and books have pointed out the deleterious effects of refined sugar consumption. A few of these are: Drs. Cheraskin and Ringsdorf, *Psychodietetics*, Bantam Books, New York, 1978; John Yudkin, M.D., *Sweet and Dangerous*, Bantam Books, New York, 1973; David Reuben, M.D., *Everything You Always Wanted to Know About Nutrition*, Avon, New York, 1979; and William Dufty, *Sugar Blues*, Warner Books, New York, 1975.
2. An informative article describing the properties, uses, and methods

of processing natural sweeteners is Richard Leviton's "A Shopper's Guide to Sweeteners," *East/West Journal*, May 1986.
3. Paavo Airola, Ph.D., N.D., *Rejuvenation Secrets from Around the World*, Health Plus, Phoenix, Ariz., 1977, pp. 42–46.

APPENDIX E

■

QUESTIONS AND ANSWERS

The following are some of the questions I have been asked that have not been specifically discussed in the text. Since many of these questions are of general interest, I include them here.

I'm from Texas. People can become immune to snake bites by being bitten by snakes. Isn't immunization based upon the same principle?

You can become desensitized to—sometimes called "building a tolerance for"—a toxin by gradually increasing your exposure to it. For instance, when a person first starts to smoke it usually makes him/her sick, but gradually the body adjusts. Could you honestly say that person is healthier?

What we are talking about here—and throughout this book—is establishing "broad spectrum" immunity rather than merely disease specific immunity.

I don't want my children immunized, but our state has a compulsory immunization law. How do I get out of it?

This is the most commonly asked question. See Appendix B.

My cousin had whooping cough, and it lasted almost four months. She almost died. Wouldn't the risk of shots be better than this?

This is a two-pronged question. First, you are assuming that immunizations work, that they really do prevent the diseases for which they are given. Second, you are assuming that because someone else had a severe case of an illness, there is nothing you can do to prevent a similar occurrence except immunize. In answer to both of these, read this book. You may wish to pursue the matter further by reading some of the references I have used such as books by Drs. Airola, Buttram, Moskowitz, and Mendelsohn. Dr. Gordon Stewart said in the interview in *D.P.T.: Vaccine Roulette* that when children die of whooping cough it is because they are severely disadvantaged in some way. Evidence suggests that a healthy child, properly cared for, will not die from whooping cough nor will the disease be serious or protracted.

If you still feel uneasy about not having your child "protected," I would suggest you see a homeopathic doctor. He can give your child oral immunizing agents that are harmless.

Immunizations do have an effect. They work. How do you explain that commercial chickens that were dying by the thousands from some disease caused by the terrible conditions under which they were kept are no longer dying of it because of a vaccine that was developed?

Go back to principle. If you have an undesirable condition and you make it disappear without correcting the cause, watch out. It will surface later in another form and one that is usually more serious or debilitating. In the healing arts we call this the progression from acute to chronic to degenerative disease. Artificially raised animals are usually slaughtered before the chronic or degenerative form of the disease is visible. We eat the diseased flesh and become diseased ourselves. Some of the hormones used in feeding commercial animals, for instance, have been linked to cancer in humans.

I knew a young man years ago who worked for a while cutting up chickens in a meat packing facility. He made the mistake of not wearing gloves, and he developed a painful and unsightly skin condition on his hands and forearms just from handling the meat! He told me horror stories of diseased animals in which the diseased parts were cut out and the rest cut and packaged for human consumption. Many think that practices like this contribute to our high rate of degenerative disease.

If doctors—chiropractors, naturopaths, homeopaths, herbalists, etc.—using natural methods of healing are so effective, why don't we hear about any great contributions they have made? What research has been done to demonstrate that their methods work?

I once heard a chiropractor in a public lecture say that because chiropractic does not get funds from government and big corporations, such as the pharmaceutical houses, he can't point to this or that controlled study and say this is what we found. In fact, he said, when a chiropractor goes out to practice he is learning. "Every day I am learning and discovering the remarkable benefits of chiropractic. I treat for one condition and other conditions seem to clear up in the process," he said. Other health care practitioners who use natural methods have made similar remarks. Obviously, their methods don't make money for pharmaceutical houses, surgeons, medical technicians, and manufacturers of expensive medical equipment. Hence, research in natural therapies is not financed by big moneyed interests.

Also, who are the big advertisers? Industries engaged in the manufacture of hi tech commodities which include drugs and vaccines. Advertising is the financial lifeline of the media, and stories that do not support the interests of their advertisers are not published.

But natural and holistic healing has a long and honorable history. The current interest in holistic healing, nutrition, body movement, and color and music therapies began with Pythagoras in 580 B.C., at least a century before Hippocrates. The latter carried on this tradition using herbs and diet and advocating a practice we today call chiropractic.

Another reason you don't hear about the breakthroughs in natural healing is that they are, for the most part, individual and anecdotal. Central to the philosophy of holistic natural healing such as homeopathy is the idea that patients are people, not numbers, things, or mindless bodies. Illnesses are not entities that can be separated from the people who have them; hence, assembly line treatment as practiced by most of mainstream medicine has no place. Again, this latter style of health care is where the money is.

Until someone can figure out how to make substantial profits by selling such things as sunshine, fresh air, pure water, natural food and herbs, exercise, positive thinking, and self-sufficiency, you're going to have to be content with anecdotal evidence, and there is plenty of that.

Are you saying that vaccinations exist because drug companies and doctors make a profit from them?

There is no doubt that vaccines are big business. The research and administration of vaccines employs tens of thousands of people in drug companies, private research laboratories, universities, state health departments, public health clinics, the FDA, the CDC (Centers for Disease Control), hospitals, and doctors' offices. States obtain federal grants to hire additional personnel in their health departments to implement mass immunization programs.

The CDC estimates that the eight major vaccines distributed in the United States in 1981 generated more than $300 million for the drug industry.[1] For an industry which grosses sales in the tens of billions of dollars a year this is not a significant amount of money. What is significant, though, is the mind-set that is promoted by this ritual. It is this mind-set that makes the money. It is a mind-set that sees disease as a frightening, foreign invader, an implacable enemy whose mysteries can only be fathomed by men versed in a specific technology and whose defeat depends entirely upon their ministrations.

Most medical doctors, being products of the system they serve, are probably sincere. They probably believe in what they are doing; however, I have read of studies and have heard of individual cases where doctors refuse to give their own children some of the immunizations they give to other children. You have to remember medical doctors are under a lot of pressure from their local medical society. If they don't conform, they could be ousted or, at least, censured. How much their sincerity is distorted by pressure to conform is anybody's guess.

Do you know what Edgar Cayce said about immunizations?

One of the most valuable and interesting features of the Cayce health readings is their holistic nature. In an editorial of the *Journal of the American Medical Association* (March 16, 1979), John P. Callan, M.D., said, "The roots of present-day holism probably go back 100 years to the birth of Edgar Cayce in Hopkinsville, Kentucky." So when we read an Edgar Cayce reading we must remember that we are reading a message that addresses the consciousness of the person requesting the reading. Cayce once used the term "castor oil consciousness." Is it too much to use the term "immunization consciousness"; and wouldn't his answers be somewhat different for someone with a strong immunization consciousness than for someone with a different consciousness?

I have read quite a number of the Cayce readings on immunizations and the only consistency I can find is that he never recommended them as part of a health care program. His advice was always in answer to a question about some immunization or immunizations in general. Generally he said that vaccines should not be mixed; give only one at a time. Sometimes he told parents to wait until a particular age to have it done, frequently saying that if the body were kept in an alkaline condition by the addition of carrots, celery, lettuce, and the like each day, there would be no need for immunizations. Sometimes he told people to stay away from them, particularly, the smallpox vaccination. One parent who had given her child the diphtheria and whooping cough injections asked if they were "detrimental to the body" and, if so, what could be done. Cayce advised her to "do the things that would be in keeping with making the normal conditions, overcoming the harm already done." He advised among other things better eliminations and circulation. (3172–2) I know one case of a child who had a vaccine injury and he prescribed a purification regime and she recovered.

An excerpt from a Cayce reading sheds a revealing light on this entire discussion: "Many times has the evolution of the earth reached the stage of development as it has today, and then [sunk] again, to rise again in the next development. Some along one line, some along others, for often we find the higher branches of co-called learning destroys itself in the seed it produces in man's development, *as we have in the medical forces* . . . as we have in some forms of spiritual forces, as we have in forms of destructive forces of the various natures."

(900–70) (Italics mine)

NOTE

1. Harris L. Coulter and Barbara Loe Fisher, *DPT: A Shot in the Dark*, Harcourt Brace Jovanowich, New York, 1985, p. 406.

APPENDIX F

■

"I HAVE A DREAM"

I have a dream that one day we will have temple-spas throughout the country where people will go to renew their spirits, nourish their minds, and regenerate their bodies. These temple-spas will be surrounded by gardens, fragrant with the scent of herbs and flowers, with pathways leading to nearby woods and meadows. Certain areas of the temple-spa will be set aside for specialized activities, each contributing to attunement to the Universal: (1) natural therapies such as music, color, massage, manipulation, and hydro- and helio-therapies; (2) body movement such as dancing, swimming, yoga, and Tai Chi; (3) programs such as music, drama and lecture/discussion; (4) libraries for reading and research; (5) creative activities such as working with arts and crafts; (6) working with nature through gardening or study; and (7) turning within through prayer and meditation. A common denominator of the temple-spa experience will be individualized therapeutic programs and a large, windowed cafeteria serving fresh, whole, unadulterated, organically grown food and pure, unpolluted water.

These temple-spas will be as much a part of our national life as hospitals and churches are today. An impossible dream? So was the airplane and the telephone, in fact, most of what we call modern civilization. Progress begins with impossible dreams; except, this time around, the impossible dream must be of a different nature, must move us in a different direction if we are to survive into the 21st century. The new direction will be towards health, wholeness, and harmony both within and without—ourselves and our world. This is the peace we are seeking.

INDEX